The Clinical Pharmacology of Anti-Inflammatory Agents

The Clinical Pharmacology of Anti-Inflammatory Agents

Peter M. Brooks
University of Sydney, New South Wales, Australia

Walter F. Kean
McMaster University Medical School, Hamilton, Ontario, Canada

and

W. Watson Buchanan
McMaster University Medical School, Hamilton, Ontario, Canada

Taylor & Francis
London and Philadelphia
1986

UK Taylor & Francis Ltd, 4 John St., London WC1N 2ET

USA Taylor & Francis Inc., 242 Cherry St., Philadelphia
PA 19106–1906

British Library Cataloguing in Publication Data

Brooks, Peter M.
The clinical pharmacology of anti-inflammatory agents.
1. Anti-inflammatory agents
I. Title II. Kean, Walter F.
III. Buchanan, W. Watson
615′.7 RM405

ISBN 0-85066-331-8

Library of Congress Cataloging in Publication Data is available

Cover design by Russell Beach
Typeset by Mathematical Composition Setters Ltd, Ivy Street, Salisbury
Printed in Great Britain by Taylor & Francis (Printers) Ltd, Rankine Road, Basingstoke, Hampshire RG24 0PR, UK

Contents

To our wives,
Helen, Mary and Margaret

About the authors

Peter Brooks, M.D., B.S. (Monash), F.R.A.C.P., F.A.C.R.M.
is the foundation Florance and Cope Professor of Rheumatology at the University of Sydney. He is the Head of the Department of Rheumatology at the Royal North Shore Hospital of Sydney. He first became interested in the clinical pharmacology of inflammation and its control while working at the Centre for Rheumatic Diseases, Baird Street, Glasgow, Scotland with Watson Buchanan in the early 1970s. His major research interests now include basic mechanisms of inflammation and mechanisms of action of anti-inflammatory drugs as well as psychological manifestations of chronic rheumatic diseases.

Walter F. Kean, M.D., Ch.B. (Glasgow), F.R.C.P. (C)
graduated from Glasgow University in 1972 and moved to Canada where he studied internal medicine and rheumatology before moving to McMaster University, Hamilton, Ontario in 1980. Walter Kean has a major research interest in the mechanism of action of gold-thiol complexes and the pharmacokinetics of NSAIDs in the elderly. He has edited a book on rheumatic diseases in the elderly and is coauthor of other rheumatology texts. He is presently an Associate Professor of Medicine and Co-Director of the Laboratory for Inorganic Medicine at McMaster University.

Watson Buchanan, M.D., F.R.C.P. (Glasgow, Edinburgh, and Canada), F.A.C.P.
has made a number of important contributions to rheumatology during his years as Physician-In-Charge of the Centre for Rheumatic Diseases in Glasgow where he was also Titular Professor of Medicine at the University of Glasgow, Scotland and as Professor of Medicine and Chief of Rheumatology, McMaster University, Hamilton, Ontario, Canada. Dr. Buchanan has a major interest in measurement of disease activity in inflammatory joint disease. With Dr. James A. Boyle he coauthored a textbook of Clinical Rheumatology, as well as other textbooks on multiple choice questions, clinical examination of the locomotor system and critical review of clinical trials of anti-rheumatic drugs.

Acknowledgements

We wish to thank Dr. Margaret McCredie for drawing the structural formulae and Barbara Forbes-Smith for typing the manuscript.

Introduction

Inflammation is one of the basic pathological processes producing tissue damage. It is the cause of joint destruction in the rheumatic diseases where it leads to significant pain and disability.

In this book we have attempted to review the process of inflammation and look at some of the pharmacological methods used to control the inflammatory process. Following a description of the pathogenesis of inflammation and its assessment, the different classes of anti-inflammatory and anti-rheumatic drugs are reviewed. Each chapter is concerned with a particular group of anti-inflammatory agents, reviewing their chemistry, pharmacology, toxicology and pharmacokinetics, and providing a brief description of their clinical effect.

A broad classification of anti-inflammatory, analgesic agents is shown in table 1. Pure analgesic agents, such as paracetamol (acetaminophen), codeine derivatives, pentazocine, propoxyphene and the opioids, will modulate pain perception, but do not influence inflammation. However, it is thought that many of the non-steroidal anti-inflammatory drugs (NSAIDs) may have a primary analgesic effect when used in low dose.

The largest group of anti-inflammatory analgesic agents comprises the NSAIDs. The best known of these are the salicylates, but over the last 60 years many new drugs have been produced. Although the NSAIDs share a common mechanism of action, interfering with the activity of cyclo-oxygenase and thus reducing prostaglandin formation, they have many other biochemical and immunological effects. However, some of the newer drugs seem to have a lower incidence of side-effects and may act specifically on certain inflammatory pathways.

The slow-acting anti-rheumatic drugs (SAARDs) affect the cellular aspects of inflammation. They work over a prolonged period of time and clinical responses to them are delayed. They comprise the anti-malarials, gold compounds, D-penicillamine, other thiol drugs and sulphasalazine.

Corticosteroid agents are potent inhibitors of the inflammatory response and may be given orally, by intravenous injection or by injection into inflamed areas in or around the synovial tissues.

The major immunosuppressive agents used in rheumatic disease are azathioprine, methotrexate, chlorambucil and 6-mercaptopurine. These drugs

Table 1. Anti-inflammatory analgesic agents.

Pure analgesic agents
Non-steroidal anti-inflammatory drugs (NSAIDs)
Slow-acting anti-rheumatic drugs (SAARDs)
Anti-malarials
Gold compounds
D-penicillamine and other thiol drugs
Sulphasalazine
Corticosteroids
Immunosuppressive agents
Anti-gout preparations
Colchicine
Uricosuric agents
Allopurinol

suppress cellular elements of the inflammatory response, but major side-effects are encountered with their long-term use.

Three major groups of anti-gout preparation are available including anti-inflammatory agents, such as NSAIDs or colchicine, the uricosuric agents, sulphinpyrazone and probenecid, and the xanthine-oxidase inhibitor allopurinol.

All anti-inflammatory, analgesic agents may be used alone or in combination, depending on the nature of the inflammatory response. However, owing to the complicated nature of inflammation it is likely that better control will be achieved by using a combination of drugs from different groups, particularly when they have different spectra of activity or side-effects, or drugs from within the same group.

> "Hear the rest, and you will marvel even more at the crafts and resources I've contrived. Greatest was this: in the former times if a man fell sick he had no defence against the sickness, neither healing food nor drink, nor unguent; but through the lack of drugs men wasted away, until I showed them the blending of mild simples wherewith they drive out all manner of diseases."
>
> Aeschylus (525–456 BC)

1. Inflammation

The rheumatic diseases are among some of the most common complaints affecting mankind. There are at least 150 different types of arthritis ranging from transient, post-traumatic, soft-tissue rheumatism to severe, destructive, rheumatoid arthritis. The basic pathological process in all these conditions is inflammation.

The inflammatory response is determined by a variety of factors which follow the primary event, producing immunological and pharmacological responses. These 'responses' are transferred via the body fluids (usually the blood) to the effector cells (the white cells, platelets etc.), where activation occurs. The subsequent release of a number of destructive molecules—arachidonic-acid metabolites and oxygen radicals—results in tissue damage. All stages of this process are regulated by positive- and negative-feedback loops.

The basic principles of inflammation, as they apply to rheumatic disease, are discussed in this chapter. The same principles may, however, pertain to other diseases in which inflammation plays a key role.

Inflammation in rheumatic disease is best exemplified by rheumatoid arthritis. In other types of inflammatory joint disease, such as the sero-negative spondyloarthropathies, the pathology is similar, although the initiating factor or factors may be different. In osteoarthritis the primary event would seem to be cartilage breakdown and the secondary event, mild inflammatory synovitis.

More and more evidence is being obtained to support a genetic basis for rheumatic diseases. The association of the human leucocyte antigen HLA–B27 with ankylosing spondylitis and a variety of reactive arthropathies, is now well established. Recent work has demonstrated an association between rheumatoid arthritis and a number of histo-compatibility antigens in the D-related (DR) locus of the major human histo-compatibility complex. The DR4 antigen, for example, is more prevalent in patients with rheumatoid arthritis, particularly in those who have rheumatoid factor in their serum.

Microbial factors

Although the relationship of microbial agents to rheumatoid arthritis remains hypothetical, many pyogenic bacteria, mycobacteria, fungi and viruses can multiply within the synovial cavity. Other micro-organisms may localise in the joint space (rubella) or become associated with immune complexes which are taken up by the joint (e.g., the immune complexes associated with hepatitis B). Bacteria, such as the streptococcus, may produce cross-reacting antibodies which give rise to synovitis, their cell walls acting as initiating agents in this process. Indeed, streptococcal peptido-glycans have been shown to remain within macrophages for long periods of time and are strongly arthritogenic in a variety of animal models.

Many viruses, including adenovirus and Coxsackie virus, are associated with polysynovitis. The arbovirus, Ross river virus, is carried by mosquitos and is associated with an epidemic polyarthritis and a maculo-papulo skin rash. Other viruses, such as the Epstein–Barr virus, have been accorded an aetiological role in rheumatoid arthritis. Epstein–Barr virus is particularly interesting as it is a polyclonal B-cell activator and more than 90% of adults show serological evidence of having been infected with it. However, the development of rheumatoid arthritis is complex, possibly depending on a number of viruses as well as genetic and environmental factors.

Pathology

In the normal diarthrodal joint (figure 1.1) articular cartilage covers the bone ends and the joint capsule is lined by a thin layer of synovial tissue. Articular cartilage is a dense matrix of collagen and proteoglycans containing the occasional chondrocyte. It is divided into four zones, superficial, intermediate, deep and calcified. The superficial zone is at the surface of the articular cartilage. Here, the collagen fibres are orientated at a tangent to the surface and contain little proteoglycan. In the intermediate or transitional zone the collagen fibres are randomly orientated and, in the deep or radial zone, collagen fibres are found perpendicular to the surface and fixed firmly to the sub-chondral bone plate. The collagen fibre and proteoglycan matrix retains a large amount of water and this provides the cartilage with many of its elastic properties. As the cartilage is devoid of blood vessels, chondrocytes deep in the matrix must obtain nutrients from the synovial fluid by diffusion, intermittent compression of cartilage or by active transport. Changes in the water content of cartilage lead to alterations in its elasticity and the development of degenerative joint disease. Although, in the past, it was felt that cartilage was unable to repair itself, there is evidence that the chondrocytes can proliferate and enable some healing to occur.

The synovial membrane which lines the joint capsule is made up of synovial lining cells overlying fatty and fibrous tissue. These cells, which produce hyaluronic acid, the major constituent of synovial fluid, can be classified into three different types. Type A cells (prominent Golgi apparatus, vesicles and vacuoles) have a major phagocytic (macrophage-like) function; type B cells,

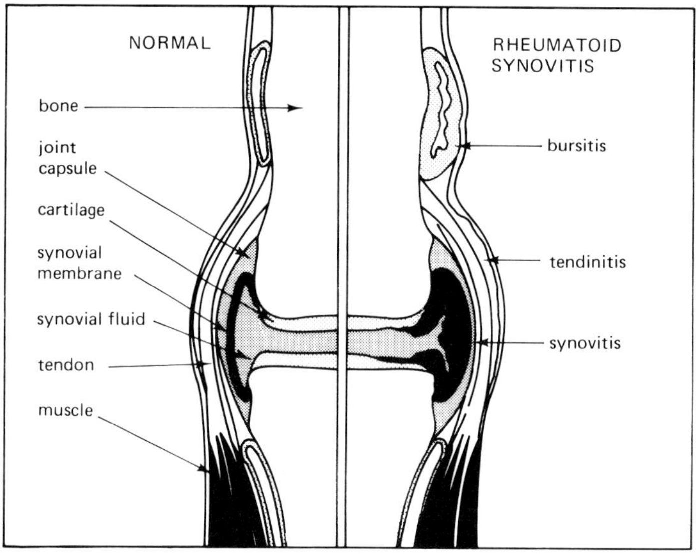

Figure 1.1. Diagram of normal and inflamed diarthrodal joint.
Adapted from *Atlas of Clinical Rheumatology*, by P. A. Dieppe, P. A. Bacon, A. N. Bamji and I. Watt (Gower Medical Publishing).

with prominent endoplasmic reticulum, act as fibroblasts; and C (or intermediate) cells have features of both fibroblast and macrophage and may represent an early stage of differentiation. The synovial lining is normally no more than three to four cells in thickness. However, some synovial blood vessels are present and the whole is surrounded by fibrous tissue and fat. The synovial membrane does not have a basement membrane and, thus, no anatomical barrier exists between the synovial fluid and synovial blood vessels.

Synovial fluid, which aids the movement of cartilage surfaces over each other during normal joint motion, is a filtrate of plasma from the sub-synovial capillaries, to which hyaluronic acid, secreted by the synovial cells, is added. Normal synovial fluid contains a few cells, a number of proteins and hyaluronic acid. Under normal conditions, large molecules such as alpha-2 macroglobulin (the principal proteinase inhibitor of plasma), fibrinogen and IgM are almost totally excluded from passing through the synovial interstitium by hyaluronic acid. However, once the joint is inflamed, this barrier breaks down and larger proteins can pass through.

In rheumatoid joint inflammation the earliest changes are seen in the small blood vessels of the sub-synovial connective tissues. These become dilated and a proliferation of vascular tissues occurs. Careful examination of the vascular endothelium reveals gaps which allow fluid and cells to leave the intravascular compartment, producing interstitial oedema. At an early stage, the blood vessels become obliterated by platelet thrombi and attract mononuclear cells.

Initially, these cells are primarily T cells, but, as the inflammatory lesion becomes chronic, the synovial cell layer proliferates, is infiltrated with chronic inflammatory cells and accumulates oedema fluid. The blood vessels in the sub-synovial layer demonstrate local and segmental changes, with venous distension, capillary obstruction and infiltration of the vessel walls by neutrophils. Fibrin is laid down in the connective tissue stroma, particularly around the small blood vessels and this sub-synovial space becomes infiltrated with lymphocytes and immunoglobulin. Lymphocyte follicles occur in the sub-synovial area and are composed mainly of T cells, although, later, plasma cells start to appear. The lymphocytes produced are in various stages of activation, but specific transitional areas occur in the synovial membrane, where over two thirds of the cells are in an activated state, and it is felt that these are the areas where antibody and mediator production are at their peak. At the junction with the articular cartilage, the proliferating synovial tissue (pannus) begins to invade the cartilage surface. The cartilage–pannus junction is the active site of cartilage destruction with lymphocytes, plasma cells and macrophages interacting with matrix and chondrocytes. Proteoglycan aggregates within the cartilage are broken up both by neutral proteinase released from the synovial cells and by chondrocytes. The small proteoglycans are then further degraded by enzymes such as cathepsin D and sulphatase. Elastase cleaves the cross-linked regions from collagen fibrils while collagenase cleaves the helical regions. The remaining collagen fragments spontaneously denature and are further metabolized by neutral proteinases and collagenolytic cathepsins. Fragments of collagen are strongly chemotactic for monocytes as well as fibroblasts. Finally, the absorption of bone mineral occurs, as osteoclasts are activated by arachidonic-acid metabolites or cytokines.

Lymphocyte infiltration

The majority of lymphocytes in the inflamed synovium are T cells. Careful histological studies have shown a marked variation in T-cell population throughout the rheumatoid synovium, but cells of the OK T4 (helper/inducer) series are seen primarily in the small lymphocyte collections, while those of the OK T8 cytotoxic drug suppressor series predominate in the active 'transitional areas'. T-cell proliferation, in these immunologically active areas, occurs as a result of macrophage interaction and leads to the secretion of a variety of biologically-active, soluble substances that stimulate antibody production by B cells.

In contrast to the large numbers of T cells, there is a small but significant number of B lymphocytes, which mediate local antibody production. Immunoglobulin synthesis occurs in the synovial tissue and large amounts of IgG and IgM, either alone or in combination, are found in the cells of the synovial lining, in the sub-synovial connective tissue, and around the synovial blood vessels. The lymphocytes of the rheumatoid synovium seem to be attracted to different antigens than the peripheral blood lymphocytes. In rheumatoid arthritis the most common immunoglobulin product is rheumatoid factor, which is directed against IgG.

The role of rheumatoid factor in the genesis of rheumatoid arthritis is still unclear. While patients with hypogammaglobulinaemia and negligible circulating IgG can develop rheumatoid arthritis, there is a strong association between the presence of serum rheumatoid factor and extra-articular manifestations of the disease. Approximately 70% of patients with rheumatoid arthritis are positive for IgM rheumatoid factor and it is likely that many patients with sero-negative disease have IgG rheumatoid factor, but that it is masked by other serum proteins. The role of genetic factors in the production of rheumatoid factor is unclear, but family studies suggest that they are important. Within the synovium high concentrations of antibody, together with low concentrations of antigen, lead to the production of intermediate-size immune complexes which fix complement and are highly immunogenic. In serum, small complexes are often formed. These are usually stable and not capable of fixing complement. However, in certain situations, large or intermediate-size complexes form and cause immune-complex-mediated vasculitis.

Macrophages

Macrophage-like cells are found in the synovial lining and in the pannus, which invades the cartilage in chronic rheumatoid arthritis. They are activated by a variety of factors, including chemicals known as cytokines, which may be released from T lymphocytes. A variety of cytokines and other inflammatory substances, such as the complement component C5a, denatured protein and collagen, may be chemotactic to macrophages, attracting them to the sites of inflammation. Once activated, the macrophages undergo a burst of metabolic activity, which may involve phagocytosis and the release of a variety of soluble mediators including neutral proteinases, such as plasminogen activator and collagenase, acid hydrolases, complement components, arachidonic-acid metabolites, and reactive metabolites of oxygen such as the superoxide radical. Oxygen radicals are also released from a variety of other cells during inflammation and play a very important role in activating enzymes, destroying proteins, and causing extensive tissue damage.

Macrophages induce vascular proliferation within inflamed connective tissues and promote fibroblast proliferation. They have a large number of surface receptors, including Fc, complement, and glycoprotein receptors, which play an important role in their anti-microbial and immunoregulatory functions. The interaction between T lymphocytes and macrophages is important to inflammation and gives credence to the theory that rheumatoid arthritis results from a delayed-type hypersensitivity reaction. Antigen-stimulated lymphocytes release cytokines which activate macrophages, but macrophages may modify antigen recognition by T lymphocytes through immune-response genes found on the macrophage membrane. In addition, macrophages may process antigen and present it to the lymphocyte, stimulating the release of cytokines.

The pannus

The pannus is vascular granulation tissue and is made up of proliferating fibroblasts, blood vessels and a variety of inflammatory cells. Three types of pannus have been described. The first is known as the cellular pannus, being synovial-like in appearance and infiltrating the cartilage with new blood vessels and perivascular mononuclear cells. Enzymes are released from the mononuclear cells and destroy the cartilage. The second type of pannus is composed of fibroblasts and monocytes, around which cartilage degradation occurs, but the third type of pannus is avascular and seems to occur as a result of tissue injury. It is composed of dense acellular fibrous tissue which may interfere with cartilage nutrition.

Polymorphonuclear leucocytes

Although polymorphonuclear leucocytes (PMN) are not found to any great extent in the synovial lining, they are the major cell in inflammatory synovial fluid. It is thought that the PMNs migrate from the intravascular compartment and are trapped in the synovial fluid. A number of chemotactic factors are released during the inflammatory process (e.g., complement components, histamine, and arachidonic-acid metabolites), which are chemotactic for human PMNs. Within the inflamed joint PMNs are involved in phagocytosis causing tissue damage by releasing large numbers of oxygen radicals and a variety of lysosomal enzymes. In addition, they can aggregate and cause microvascular occlusion within the synovial tissue, precipitating ischaemic tissue damage. The activation of PMNs is associated with the internal release of the lipoxygenase metabolite, leukotriene B4.

Platelets

The potential contribution of the platelet to inflammation and, in particular, rheumatoid arthritis, is considerable. The fact that platelets accumulate intravascularly at sites of tissue injury, and specifically within thrombosed synovial vessels, has been clearly demonstrated. However, they do tend to remain within the vascular compartment. Platelets can also adhere to other inflammatory cells, and may act as inflammatory mediators. During activation, they release serotonin, arachidonic-acid metabolites, acid hydrolases and factors which stimulate the proliferation of vascular smooth muscle cells. However, it has yet to be determined whether platelet aggregation occurs as a secondary event in inflammatory reactions or plays a more pivotal role.

Humoral factors

The cells involved in inflammation all give rise to chemical mediators which produce tissue damage.

Complement

The complement cascade (figure 1.2) comprises a series of proteins, found in normal serum. It can be activated by immune and cellular responses. Once triggered, the proteins interact in a cascade sequence that eventually leads to cell lysis. In activating this sequence, a variety of proteases are produced.

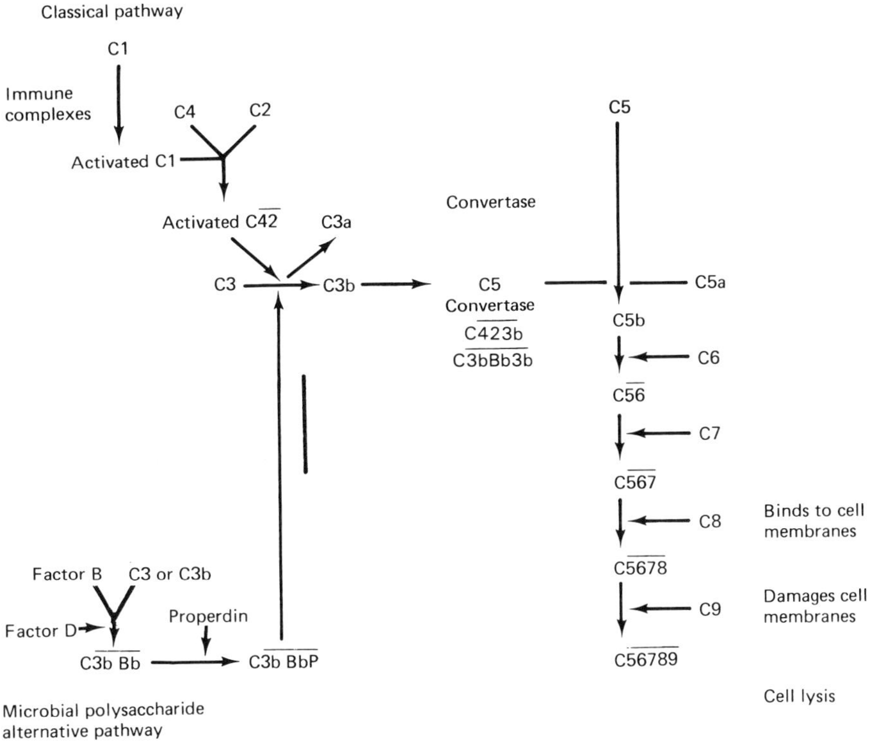

Figure 1.2. The complement cascade. The classical and alternative pathways of complement activation are shown. Activated complement proteins are marked by a horizontal bar above the sequence numbers (e.g. $\overline{C567}$).

The classical pathway is triggered by immune complexes while the alternative pathway relies on the presence of bacterial cell wall mucopolysaccharide and two proteins factors, B (the alternative pathway homologue of C2) and D (a serine protease).

The gamma globulin, properdin, although not required for activation, does improve the efficiency of the alternative pathway. C3 is the most important protein component. It acts as a link between the classical and alternative pathways and as an amplification loop to the alternative pathway by providing C3b.

Complement proteins play an important role in the production and clearance of immune complexes and in the elimination of micro-organisms, or cells altered by the invasion of micro-organisms. They can be divided into two categories—those involved in the initiation of the system, for which there are two major pathways, and those involved in mediating the effects of complement activation, which make up a final common pathway. The primary sequences, called either the classical or alternative pathway, for complement activation are shown in figure 1.2. In the classical pathway, immune complexes convert the precursor of C1 to an active enzyme. This then acts on the proteases C4 and C2 to produce an activated endopeptidase which breaks down C3. The alternative pathway is usually activated by micro-organisms, or by alterations in the cell surface membrane. Factor B joins with C3, or C3b, and is converted by the serine protease factor D, into an active complex C3Bb. This active cleavage complex is then converted by properdin into the enzyme C3bBbP which cleaves C3 to C3b. C3 convertases from both the classical and alternative pathways convert C3b into an active C5 convertase, triggering the terminal sequence of the complement pathway, involving C5, C6, C7, C8, C9 and a series of complex intermediates. The terminal protein products of the complement cascade bind to cell membranes and produce membrane damage leading to osmotic lysis of the cells.

The complement proteins have several roles to play in the development of inflammation. C4 and C2 increase vascular permeability, C3a acts as an anaphylatoxin and C3b is involved in phagocytosis, the induction of B-cell lymphocyte memory and in triggering the amplification loop of the alternative pathway. The active complexes of the terminal pathway, particularly C5, C6 and C7 bind to cell membranes, and begin to break them down. Complement activation occurs in a variety of rheumatic disorders, including systemic lupus erythematosus and severe rheumatoid arthritis with vasculitis.

Coagulation and fibrinolysis

Fibrin deposition is one of the features of chronic inflammation. It is not clear whether it is a primary or a secondary event, but products of the fibrinolytic and coagulation processes are involved in inflammatory tissue damage. The interactions of the intrinsic coagulation pathways are shown in figure 1.3. Hageman factor is a beta-globulin which binds to a variety of surfaces (cellular or otherwise) and interacts with high molecular weight kininogen and plasma thromboplastin antecedent factor (factor XI) to initiate the coagulation cascade. It does not seem to be activated by immune complexes, but may rely on crystals of uric acid and calcium pyrophosphate, or connective tissue cells which have already been damaged by immune complexes. There is increasing evidence that substances such as plasminogen activator may play an important role in maintaining the chronic nature of rheumatoid arthritis.

There are a variety of inhibitors of the coagulation enzymes. They include

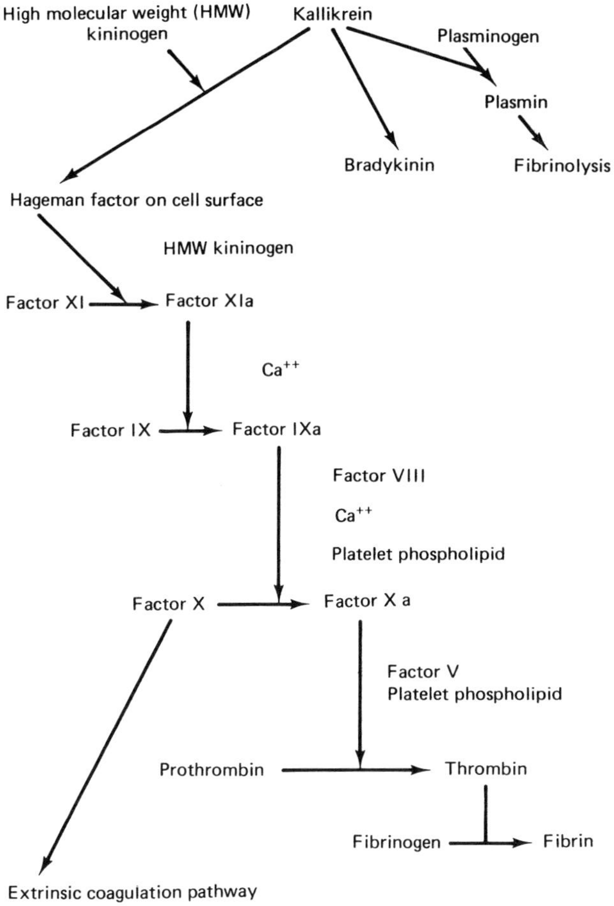

Figure 1.3. Interactions of intrinsic coagulation and fibrinolytic pathways in inflammation.

the inhibitors of the first component of complement, alpha-2-macroglobulin, alpha-1-anti-trypsin and alpha-2-anti-plasmin. These enzymes control the activation of the intrinsic coagulation pathway in inflammation and their products have a variety of other effects. Bradykinin increases vascular permeability, which leads to the further accumulation of cellular elements, and acts as a powerful pain-producing substance. Plasmin has been shown to convert a synovial pro-collagenase to a collagenase, thus augmenting connective-tissue destruction. The final deposition of fibrin, with subsequent attempted fibrinolysis, causes the accumulation of fibrin degradation products within the fibrinoid necrotic tissue seen in many of these inflammatory lesions. The exact role that these pathways play in inflammation is not clear, but they are likely to be significant.

Cytokines

When lymphocytes are activated by antigen–antibody reactions, or mitogens, they produce chemicals called lymphokines which activate a number of cells involved in the inflammatory response. There is evidence that similar chemicals are produced by macrophages and other inflammatory cells as well and, for this reason, these substances are better referred to as monokines or cytokines. The major lymphokines and the cells on which they act are shown in table 1.1. It is likely that these chemicals play a key role in the interaction between cells involved in the inflammatory process.

The behaviour of lymphocytes can be modified by cytokines. Interleukin-2 (IL-2) is important for the continuous growth of T cells, inducing proliferation and cytotoxic T-cell activity. The interferons (Ifn-alpha and Ifn-beta) have been shown to potentiate the cytolytic responses of T cells and some cytokines may be chemotactic to lymphocytes. Macrophages are activated on their exposure to cytokines, and undergo a series of well described morphological changes, increasing their size and stickiness, and the number of microvilli and phagocytic vacuoles they possess. Macrophage movement is altered too, and enhanced phagocytosis occurs, with increased activity towards microbes and tumour cells. A number of the effects produced by cytokines in the activation of macrophages are calcium-dependent. The biochemical changes that occur include increased oxygen consumption and the production of oxygen radicals, arachidonic acid metabolites (e.g., prostaglandins and leukotrienes), plasminogen activator and collagenase. Cytokines have similar effects on granulocytes, stimulating phagocytic activity, reducing migration from inflamed areas and increasing the production of reactive oxygen species. Lymphocytes produce a cytokine (osteoclast-activating factor) which leads to bone resorption and this may be dependent on products of arachidonic-acid metabolism. Vascular permeability can also be regulated by cytokine production and this again may be controlled by products of arachidonic-acid metabolism.

Cytokines are produced by proliferating cells, cause the accumulation of monocytes and granulocytes, increase vascular permeability and are involved

Table 1.1. Cytokines produced by activated lymphocytes.

Cytokine	Effector cell
Interleukin-1	Macrophage
Gamma-interferon	Lymphocyte
Macrophage migration inhibition factor	Macrophage
Macrophage-chemotaxis factor	Macrophage
Lymphocyte-mitogenic factor	Lymphocyte
Neutrophil-chemotactic factor	Neutrophils
Skin-reactive factor	Vascular endothelial cells
Osteoclast-activating factor	Osteoclasts

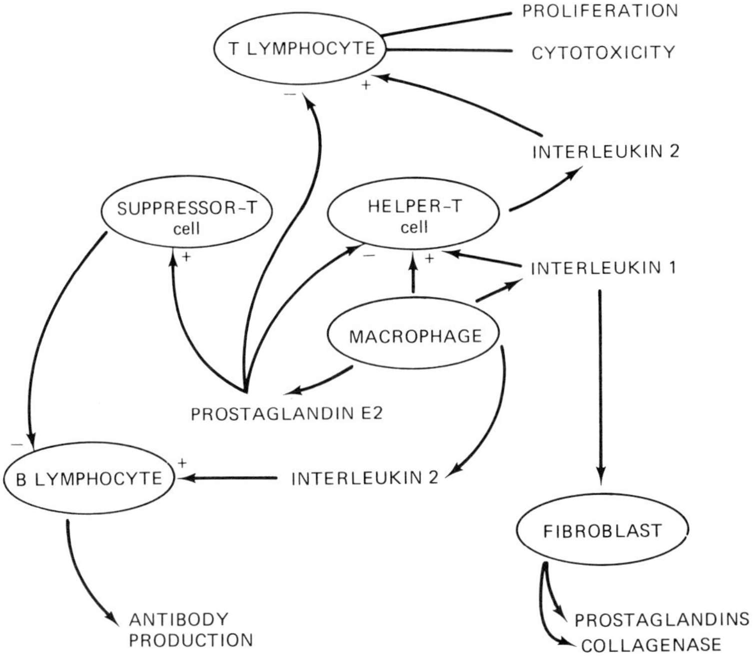

Figure 1.4. Cellular interactions in inflammation.

in lymphocyte and macrophage proliferation. Thus, there seems little doubt that the interactions between lymphocytes and macrophages are extremely important in determining the chronic nature of inflammation. During the activation of T lymphocytes the production of T-cells is triggered by the cytokine interleukin-1 (IL-1), itself produced during interaction with the antigen-presenting macrophage. The activated T cells stimulate B cells to divide giving rise to daughter blast cells with surface receptors for B-cell growth factor. B-cell growth factor stimulates B cells to mature and produce antibody. Other activated T cells produce IL-2, which stimulates the proliferation of cytotoxic T cells. The interactions occurring between lymphocyte sub-populations, fibroblasts and macrophages are shown in figure 1.4. The prostaglandins and leukotrienes produced by the macrophages can both stimulate and inhibit lymphocytes. The interactions between arachidonic-acid metabolites, cytokines and cells involved in inflammation are, thus, vitally important. It appears that cytokines act not only as effectors of the cellular immune response but also play an essential role in regulating it once it occurs.

Lysosomal enzymes

The lysosomal enzymes are hydrolases synthesized by the endoplasmic reticulum of PMNs and macrophages. Within the cell the enzymes are collected together and stored in organelles surrounded by a single membrane (lysosome). When released from their organelles, by breaches in the membrane, these enzymes break down connective tissues, including proteoglycan and collagen. The major lysosomal enzymes are collagenase, elastase and the cathepsins. Lysosomal enzymes may be active at acid pH (acid proteinases) or at neutral or slightly alkaline pH (neutral proteinases). Some are dependent for their activity on metals (e.g., copper and iron complexes) and are known as the metallo-proteinases. A variety of anti-proteinases exist within synovial fluid such as alpha-1-anti-trypsin and alpha-2-macroglobulin, both of which inhibit lysosomal-enzyme activity. The secretion of lysosomal enzymes occurs after cellular activation or during phagocytosis. Proteinases have been described in lymphocytes, monocytes, PMNs and platelets. Lysosomal enzymes are found in synovial fluid and in cartilage, particularly at the pannus–cartilage junction. There seems little doubt that they play a major role in cartilage destruction, possibly due to the fact the naturally occurring inhibitors of collagenase are excluded from the area by the advancing pannus. Lysosomal enzymes can interact with other inflammatory mediators such as the complement and coagulation systems. However, a variety of anti-inflammatory drugs including chloroquine and gold may stabilize the lysosomal membranes and prevent enzyme release.

Arachidonic-acid metabolites

The prostaglandins, thromboxanes and leukotrienes are biologically-active substances derived from the fatty acids of the cell membrane. Phospholipids in the cell membrane are converted by phospholipase to arachidonic acid. Arachidonic acid is then oxidized by two major pathways as shown in figure 1.5. The cyclo-oxygenase pathway produces stable prostaglandins, prostacyclins and thromboxanes. Most of these compounds are rapidly broken down to inactive metabolites, but those that are active produce a variety of inflammatory effects. Thromboxane A2 is a potent vasoconstrictor and platelet aggregator, while prostaglandins E2 and F2, and the prostacyclins, cause vasodilation. These compounds inhibit platelet and neutrophil aggregation by increasing the concentration of cAMP within the cells. While most prostaglandins are pro-inflammatory, prostaglandins of the E series can act in an anti-inflammatory role, possibly by increasing cAMP concentrations and inhibiting enzyme release from lymphocytes, monocytes, and PMNs.

Recently the lipoxygenase pathways have been described which lead to the production of a series of products known as leukotrienes. During the production of leukotrienes oxygen radicals are released which play a major role in tissue damage. The various cell types have different lipoxygenase enzymes—12-lipoxygenase being found in platelets, 15-lipoxygenase in T lymphocytes and 5-lipoxygenase in PMNs. Many of the products of these pathways still have to be characterized. In the 5-lipoxygenase pathway,

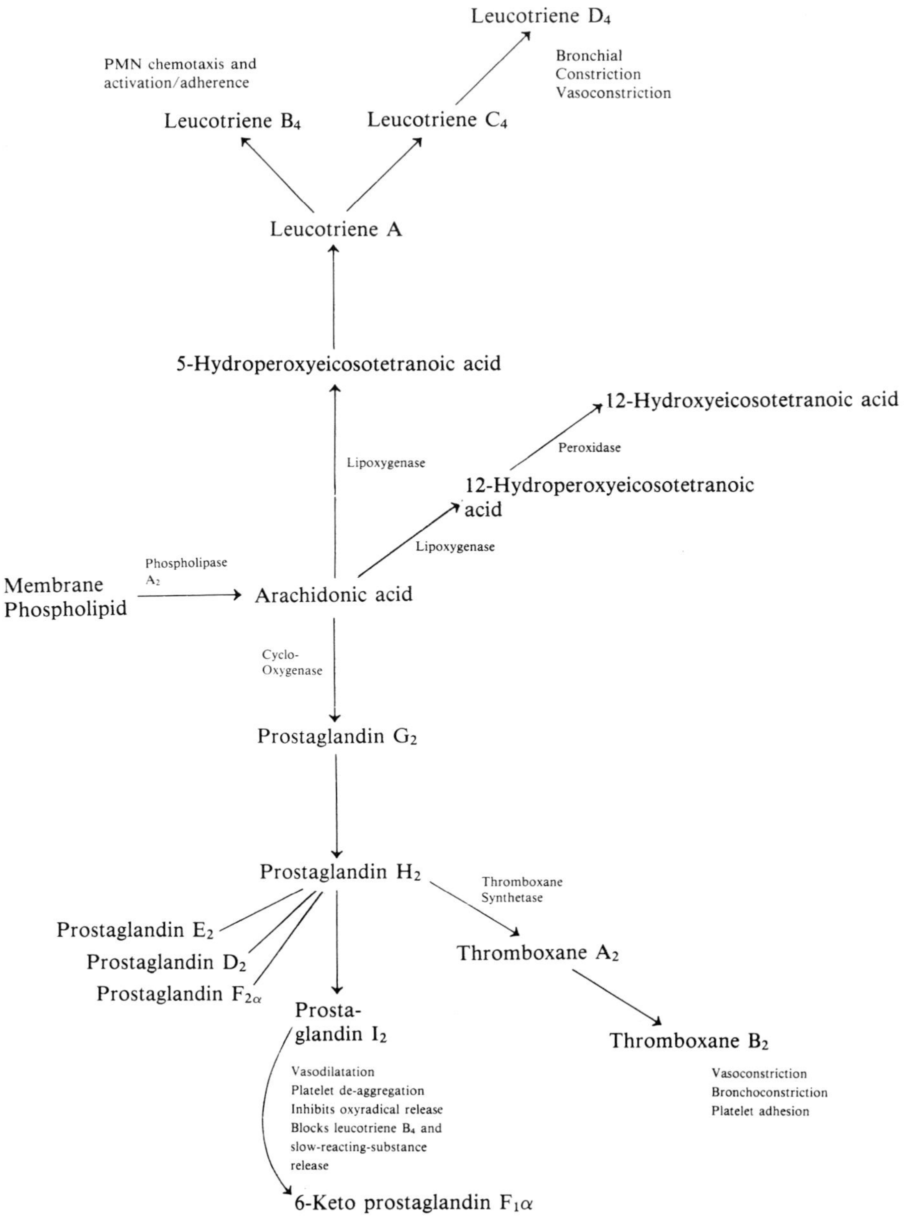

Figure 1.5. Pathways of arachidonic-acid metabolism.

leukotriene A4 is rapidly converted to leukotriene B4. This has no direct effect on blood vessels or tissues, but is a potent activator of PMNs. PMNs adhere to each other and to endothelial surfaces, thus tissue damage may be produced by sluggish circulation. Leukotreines C4 and D4, constituting the slow reacting substance of anaphylaxis, are produced by basophils and macrophages. They cause bronchoconstriction, and increased vascular permeability, particularly from the post-capillary venule.

Prostaglandins and leukotrienes act in concert during the inflammatory process and can modulate the effects of each other. The current NSAIDs have their major affect on cyclo-oxygenase, but some of the newer agents may well interfere with lipoxygenase metabolism as well. Although it has been suggested that by blocking the cyclo-oxygenase pathway, arachidonate metabolism is shunted down the lipoxygenase pathway, there is little evidence to support this hypothesis. Indeed, a great deal of work is required before the actions and interactions of the arachidonic metabolites are understood and the role that they play in inflammatory responses clarified.

Reactive-oxygen species

A free radical is defined as any species capable of independent existence having one or more unpaired electrons. The superoxide and hydroxyl radical are examples. Singlet oxygen and hydrogen peroxide can participate in reactions leading to free radical formation. These reactive oxygen species increase vascular permeability, degrade hyaluronic acid, increase PMN adhesion to the endothelium of capillaries and cause the peroxidation of lipids within cell membranes. This leads to cell lysis and death and is intimately involved with the generation of arachidonic-acid metabolites. Oxygen-radical generation occurs at the same time as the respiratory burst of PMNs during phagocytosis. The oxygen radicals are bactericidal, but cause inflammatory damage as well. A number of natural defences exist against oxygen free radicals, including the enzyme superoxide dismutase, the glutathione- and catalase-enzyme systems, vitamin E and transition metals or metallo-proteins, such as iron and ceruloplasmin. Free-radical-induced injury may occur in the extracellular spaces following their release from cells or cell membranes. Both liposomes and cellular membranes can be disrupted by free radicals and the products of radical-induced lipid peroxidation can themselves be toxic. More important, they are much more stable than oxygen radicals, and, therefore, capable of producing general damage. Intracellular organelles can be damaged by oxygen radicals and the DNA altered. This suggests that free-oxygen radicals may play a role in carcinogenesis as well as drug toxicity and inflammation. It seems likely that they are involved in the initiation of cell damage during inflammation, as well as later stages, when the products of activated inflammatory cells produce further tissue destruction. In rheumatoid arthritis, iron is found in the synovial membrane as ferritin and its presence early in the disease has

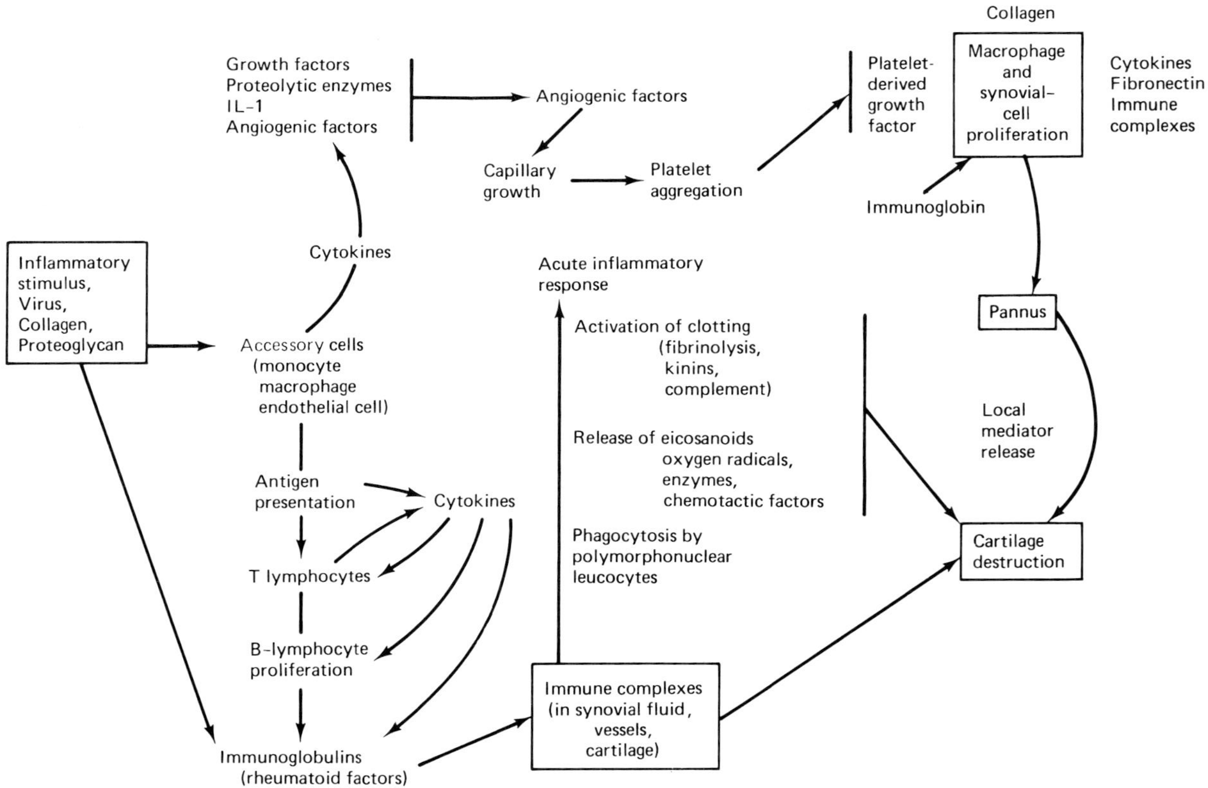

Figure 1.6. Schema of joint destruction in rheumatoid arthritis after Harris E. D., 1985, Pathogenesis of rheumatoid arthritis, in *Textbook of Rheumatology*, edited by W. N. Kelley, E. D. Harris Jr, S. Ruddy, C. B. Sledge (W. B. Saunders), p. 887.

been associated with a poor prognosis. It is possible that oxygen-radical formation is catalysed by the abundant non-protein bound iron and by the fact that synovial fluid has little superoxide dismutase or catalase activity. Iron administration to patients with rheumatoid arthritis has been associated with disease exacerbation, but the use of iron chelators has not been followed by a dramatic suppression of inflammation, although these agents are still of therapeutic interest.

Summary

Many cells and mediators take part in the inflammatory response. However, we are uncertain what the initiating factor is and what causes chronic inflammation. The major cells involved are the lymphocytes, macrophages, and PMNs, but other cellular elements, such as platelets and plasma cells, play a key role. Alterations in the microcirculation, with vasodilatation, an increase in vascular permeability and new vessel formation in the invading pannus, result in the transport of cells and mediators to the sites of tissue destruction. The role of platelets and the activation of the kinin system and the coagulation cascade may also be important in inflammation. Products of arachidonic-acid metabolism are pivotal to tissue destruction, in a large part due to the associated release of reactive-oxygen molecules which mediate tissue injury.

A variety of chemo-attractants are produced by inflammatory cells, including products of the complement cascade and cytokines, and the study of these chemicals is extremely important in determining how the chronic, inflammatory cells interact. Lysosomal enzymes play an important role in tissue destruction after the release from inflammatory cells and their balance with naturally occurring anti-proteinases, such as alpha-2-macroglobulins and alpha-1-anti-trypsin, has to be considered. A schema for tissue destruction in inflammation is shown in figure 1.6 and it can be seen that the drugs used to treat inflammation act at various points in the inflammatory cascade. The NSAIDs affect mediators of inflammation, such as the cyclo-oxygenase products and kinins. This may lead, indirectly, to a reduction in the production of oxygen radicals. The SAARDs act on the cellular mechanisms of inflammation. Gold compounds inhibit the phagocytic activity of macrophages and PMNs, stabilize lysosomal membranes and interfere with the production of prostaglandins. D-Penicillamine acts on metal chelation, and various enzyme systems, reduces serum immunoglobulin levels and has a direct effect on lymphocyte function and neutrophil chemotaxis. Recent studies suggest that it may also stimulate naturally occurring anti-oxidant materials which scavenge free-oxygen radicals. The anti-malarial drugs chloroquine and hydroxychloroquine are potent stabilizers of lysosomal membranes, but also reduce protein synthesis from cells and may inhibit prostaglandin and IL-1 production. Glucocorticoids inhibit the accumulation of cells in areas of inflammation and reduce the metabolic activity of macrophages and lymphocytes. They inhibit the release of arachidonic acid from phospholipids as well, and, hence, reduce the production of both prostaglandins and leukotrienes. The immunosuppressive agents azathioprine, methotrexate, cyclophosphamide and chlorambucil interfere with cellular aspects of inflammation by acting directly on cell function.

As the process of inflammation is so complex, it is unlikely that a single drug will have much effect. Therefore, it is to be hoped that a greater understanding of the pathways of inflammation will make the development of more specific drugs, for use in rheumatoid arthritis, a reality. In the following chapters the clinical pharmacology of the anti-inflammatory drugs is discussed.

Further reading

Allison, A. C., 1984, Role of macrophage activation in the pathogenesis of chronic inflammation and its pharmacological control. *Advances in Inflammation Research*, **7** 201–221.

Halliwell, B. and Gutteridge, J. M. C., 1984, Oxygen toxicity, oxygen radicals. Transition metals and disease. *Biochemical Journal*, **219**, 1–14.

Hanson, J. M., Rumjanek, V. M. and Morley, J., 1982, Mediators of cellular immune reactions. *Pharmacology and Therapeutics*, **17**, 165–198.

Lewis, D. H. and Del Maestro, R. editors, 1980, *Free Radicals in Medicine and Biology. Acta Physiologica Scandinavica* (Supplement 492).

Lewis, R. A. and Austen, K. F., 1984, The biologically active leukotrienes. *Journal of Clinical Investigation*, **73**, 889–897.

Weissmann, G., 1983, Pathways of arachidonate oxidation to prostaglandins and leukotrienes. *Seminars in Arthritis and Rheumatism*, **13** (supplement 1), 123–129.

Zvaifler, N. J., 1984, Immunopathology of inflammatory diseases: rheumatoid arthritis as an example. *Advances In Inflammation Research*, **7**, 1–11.

2. Assessing anti-inflammatory agents

The different classes of anti-inflammatory and anti-rheumatic drugs produce a variety of effects on *in-vitro* systems, animal models of inflammation and patients. In this chapter, the methods of assessing these drugs will be discussed.

Analgesics

Analgesic drugs have little effect on cellular mechanisms of inflammation, but may interfere with prostaglandin production, particularly in the central nervous system (CNS). The role that prostaglandin mechanisms have in the production of pain is not clear, but the analgesic effect of paracetamol is probably due in part to inhibition of prostaglandin biosynthesis in the brain. The narcotic analgesics work entirely at a neurological level, affecting either the processing of pain sensation in the brain or the entry of pain stimuli to the dorsal column of the spinal cord. There are a number of animal models that can be used to assess the effects of analgesics. These are shown in table 2.1.

Table 2.1. Animal models for assessing anti-inflammatory and anti-rheumatic drugs.

Anti-inflammatory	
Ultraviolet erythema	
Carrageenan oedema	
Kaolin-induced oedema	
Capillary permeability	
Urate-induced inflammation	
Adjuvant arthritis	Acute
	Chronic
Granuloma inhibition in cellulose or	
Cotton sponge placed subcutaneously	
Analgesic	
Acetylcholine-induced writhing	
Inflamed foot	
Mobility	
Anti-pyretic	
Yeast fever	
Pyrogen-induced fever	

Table 2.2. Clinical measurements of pain/analgesia.

Subjective
Pain threshold
Pain tolerance
Visual analogue scale
Ordinal pain scale
Verbal response
Stimulus matching
Objective
Skin conductance
Plasma cortisol
Urinary catecholamine excretion
Serum non-esterified fatty acid
Serum beta-lipoprotein
Pulmonary vital capacity
Cortical-evoked responses

Clinically, pain can be measured in a number of different ways, but it must be appreciated that pain itself is a complex, made up of the pain stimulus, the nociceptive response of the pain fibres and the pain sensation as appreciated by the brain, which may then be modified by the patient in terms of suffering and reaction. The duration and intensity of the initial stimulus may modify pain response also. A reproducible painful stimulus can be obtained by electrical stimulation, radiant heat, the application of cold water or the use of a pressure algometer. The pain sensation can be measured by a variety of methods as shown in table 2.2. Subjective measurements such as pain threshold, pain tolerance and suffering can be measured using a number of scales or verbal responses. It has also been possible to match clinical pain to other variable stimuli or to express it as a proportion of a standard painful stimulus. Several objective measures of pain which reflect the biochemical or physiological changes induced by a painful stimulus have also been described. A variety of clinical pain models exist, but any study making use of them must be carefully designed, to incorporate the double-blind, random allocation of patients and identical appearance of study medications, in order to ensure validity. If these criteria are adhered to, the clinical assessments made will be relevant to the study of the analgesic effects of anti-inflammatory and anti-rheumatic drugs.

Non-steroidal anti-inflammatory drugs

The major effects of NSAIDs *in vitro* are in the reduction of prostaglandin production in a variety of cells, including bovine and ram seminal vesicles, rheumatoid synovial cells and PMNs. In addition, they reduce the aggregation of platelets induced by adenosine diphosphate, noradrenalin and collagen, in a dose-related manner, inhibit leucocyte adherence to glass slides and reduce neutrophil chemotaxis towards casein or other attractants. Superoxide production by PMNs is inhibited by a variety of NSAIDs, as is lymphocyte responsiveness to a variety of mitogens. Complement-mediated cell lysis is reduced by some NSAIDs and, in intact animals or whole organs, they will reduce prostaglandin production from a variety of perfused organs, including guinea pig lung and cat spleen. NSAIDs stabilize lysosomal membranes in a number of tissues, including rat liver, and inhibit the release of enzymes such as acid phosphatase or aryl sulphatase.

A variety of animal models have been used to demonstrate the anti-inflammatory effects of NSAIDs (table 2.1). These models show that NSAIDs will reduce cellular infiltration and the fluid phase of inflammation. However, variation is often seen between different models with the same drug, since they tend to reflect different aspects of the inflammatory response. The standard laboratory measures of inflammatory activity, such as the erythrocyte-sedimentation rate (ESR), C-reactive protein and other acute-phase reactants, are not significantly affected by NSAIDs. On the other hand the essential amino acid L-tryptophan is displaced from its serum-albumin binding sites such that there is an increase in free tryptophan, the concentration of which is low in rheumatoid arthritis. The number of free sulphydryl groups is also reduced in patients with rheumatoid arthritis and NSAIDs will increase their serum concentration towards normal, possibly increasing their reactitivity as well. However, NSAIDs do not have any effect on the immunological markers of disease activity such as rheumatoid factor or immunoglobulin level.

The clinical measures of disease activity used to assess drug therapy in arthritis are shown in table 2.3. The principal components used to measure NSAID activity are pain, stiffness, swelling and their consequences. Pain can be measured by a number of different methods, but the most popular employed in rheumatology is self assessment using the visual-analogue scale. This scale takes the form of a line, conventionally 10 cm in length, representing a continuum of pain, with the ends of the line defining the extremes of pain (no pain or severe pain, respectively). Patients mark the line to record pain severity. It has been shown that patients can determine 21 'just-noticeable differences' in pain, from no pain to maximum pain. The design of the visual-analogue scale is important, and, while vertical or horizontal scales have been used, it seems likely that errors occur more frequently with a vertical scale and that the reproducibility of the scale may vary along its length. If descriptions of pain are marked at intervals along the line, a clustering of scores tends to occur around them, converting the, scale to a graphic-rating scale with a loss of sensitivity. With careful instruction most patients can measure pain on a visual-analogue scale. Furthermore, it has been shown that in clinical trials, rheumatoid arthritis patients benefit from being given access to their previous scores.

Pain relief has been recommended as a measure of NSAID activity, but has not gained wide acceptance in clinical trials. The perception of pain in patients depends on a number of factors, including age, anxiety, past experience and

Table 2.3. Measures of disease activity in arthritis.

Clinical	
Pain —	Visual analogue
	Interval
	Descriptive
Pain relief	
Join count (painful/tender)	
Joint count (swollen)	
Signal joint assessment	
Grip strength	
Duration of morning stiffness	
Joint circumference	
Range of motion	
Functional assessment	
Global assessment by patient	
Global assessment by physician	
Composite indices	
Haematological	
Haemoglobin	
Erythrocyte-sedimentation rate	
Platelet count	
Eosinophilia	
Biochemical	
Protein concentration	
Immunoglobulin	
C-Reactive protein	
Haptoglobin	
Fibrinogen	
Ferritin	
Sulphydryl group	
Immunological	
Rheumatoid factor	
Complement	
Radiological	
Radionuclide	
Thermography	

interaction between the subject and the observer. Some of these factors might be important, particularly in long-term studies, but the simple measurement of pain, on a visual-analogue scale, produces surprisingly robust, sensitive and reproducible results that seem to relate reasonably well to other measures of disease activity. When using a visual-analogue scale, great care must be taken to standardize the time of measurement and the form of words used for all enquiries. A simple 10 cm horizontal line, marked with terminal descriptors, should be used and adequate time allowed for an explanation of how to use it. With these guidelines, significant differences in pain can be shown, between NSAIDs and a placebo in patients with rheumatic conditions.

Joint tenderness and swelling are some of the most reliable clinical parameters of joint inflammation. Several methods exist for scoring the number of joints involved, such as them enumerating the number of painful or swollen joints, or performing an articular index. A number of articular indices have been described, but each prescribes a certain score to clinically active joints according to whether there is pain on passive movement, tenderness on pressure or inflammatory swelling. In patients with widespread joint involvement a sequential assessment of a small number of active (or so called signal) joints may provide a better measure of efficacy of anti-rheumatic therapy. One of the most widely accepted articular indices is that described by Ritchie and her colleagues. It is based on the summation of joint responses after firm digital pressure. The responses are recorded as 0, the patient has no tenderness, +1, the patient says it is painful, +2, the patient says it is painful and winces, and +3, the patient says it is painful, winces and withdraws the limb. Tenderness in some joints such as the cervical spine, hip joint, talocalcaneal and metatarsal joints is elicited by passive movement and a number of joints such as the metacarpophalangeal, and proximal interphalangeal joints are treated as single units. The maximum Ritchie index is 78 and the score obtained has been shown to reflect changes in joint inflammation and clear differences between NSAIDs and placebo in short-term trials. The basic criteria for an articular index of joint tenderness are that it should be simple to perform, highly reproducibile and show changes when the patient has an exacerbation and/or relief of symptoms, as, for example, in a flare of disease or when anti-inflammatory medication is prescribed. The Ritchie articular index would seem to fulfil these criteria and can be performed by non-medical personnel within about three minutes. It has recently been recommended by the European League Against Rheumatism Standing Committee on International Clinical Studies.

Morning stiffness is another major clinical manifestation of inflammatory joint disease. However, there is a problem with measuring this parameter since there is no precise definition of stiffness and many patients are unable to separate stiffness from pain. Some objective methods have been developed, but these usually require special apparatus and are applicable to certain joints only. Nevertheless, morning stiffness can be measured either by recording its duration or by assessing its severity using visual-analogue or graphic-rating scales. NSAIDs reduce both the duration and severity of morning stiffness.

The grip strength of the hand reflects a number of different aspects of joint disease including pain, stiffness and loss of function. A variety of instruments including spring dynamometers, torquometers, and strain gauges have been used in an effort to improve the measurement of this parameter, but have not proved to be any better than the Davis bag or sphygmomanometer cuff. In general, grip strength is relatively stable, but diurnal variation has been noted in normal subjects and in patients with rheumatoid arthritis. Measurements of grip strength have been shown to relate to those of the Ritchie articular index of joint tenderness and a functional index for the upper limbs. Recently, the use of an electronic apparatus capable of calculating several parameters of grip, including power, work and maximum grip strength, has been described. It has been suggested that these measurements provide a better discrimination between NSAIDs and placebo than maximum grip-strength measurements alone.

The measurement of joint circumference has also been shown to reflect the degree of inflammation and the efficacy of NSAIDs in reducing it. Swelling of the proximal interphalangeal joints can be measured by jeweller's rings, and plastic spring gauges or arthrocircameters. These methods are reproducible from day-to-day and week-to-week in patients with stable rheumatoid arthritis, but it is important to realize that a reduction in joint circumference can only occur in those with swelling of the soft tissue and that this reduces the usefulness of this measurement in assessing the anti-inflammatory activity of drugs in clinical trials. Nevertheless, the swelling of other joints, such as the knee, has been shown to decrease with NSAID therapy and to correlate with other parameters of disease activity.

Limitation of movement of a joint, or set of joints, may occur on either active or passive motion and may reflect pain or a mechanical abnormality. The American Academy of Orthopedic Surgeons has provided figures for the range of motion of peripheral joints in normal subjects, but this measure has proved of limited value in assessing sequential changes with drug therapy. The range of movement of certain joints, particularly the knee and the finger joints, can be assessed using a simple goniometer which measures the range of motion in degrees. Spinal movement and chest expansion can be used as measures of disease activity in the sero-negative spondyloarthropathies. Spinal mobility can be assessed in flexion, extension and rotation using instruments such as the Dunham spondylometer and inclinometer, which works on a pendulum principle, or by simple objective clinical methods requiring no more than a tape measure. Indirect measures such as the finger tip to floor distance and occiput to wall distance may also reflect sequential change in spinal movement. Measurement of chest expansion can be made by tape measure or specially adapted calipers. In patients who have a major inflammatory component to their spondyloarthropathy, but who are without fixed deformity, small, but significant, changes can often be seen with NSAID and physical therapies.

Pain and swelling in a joint tend to lead to loss of function, and although disability is probably the most important feature of chronic rheumatic disease, its measurement has proved difficult. The timing of certain movements such as a 50-foot walk has gained some acceptance in clinical trials, but there are few studies to validate its reproducibility. Early functional assessments depended on the ability to perform certain tasks with or without assistance. Indexes of disability can be numerically scored and significant improvement shown with major interventions such as reconstructive surgery. Recently, a number of questionnaires have been developed to measure functional ability, quality-of-life and health status in patients with chronic joint disease. The perfect functional assessment or quality-of-life instrument has not been designed, but the instruments in use have provided data that appear to relate well to other measures of disease activity, such as mobility and pain. It has been shown that some categories of function, such as self care, physical activity/inability, pain and role activity, are more important than others, but these may be difficult to measure because of a dependence on such things as patient expectations, goals and other social supports. It is likely that functional indices and quality-of-life scales are important in assessing the effects of therapeutic intervention, but great care must be taken in choosing the appropriate instrument to assess these particular measures. The instrument chosen in any particular situation will be determined by the purpose and duration of the study, the statistical properties of the instrument, the type of intervention that is planned, logistical considerations and the target population. By tailoring the instruments to the particular study population, function and quality-of-life measures may prove to be powerful tools for assessing the effects of therapeutic intervention in chronic joint disease.

Radionuclides have been used in a number of ways to quantify joint inflammation. These may be administered intra-articularly, and the rate of clearance from the joint determined, or intravenously, and the accumulation over a joint (or joints) assessed. The clearance of xenon-133 following intra-articular injection has been shown to provide an indirect measure of the rate of synovial blood flow. The clearance of xenon from the joint correlates with clinical assessments of disease activity, but has not been widely used in clinical trials. The accumulation of radionuclide around the joints, after intravenous injection, can be monitored by a display scintiscan or camera, or by determining peak counts. The most commonly used intravenous isotopes are technetium compounds with the pertechnetate ($^{99}Tc^{m}O_4$) being more useful than the phosphate compounds, which tend to be absorbed around cartilage or bone, reflecting changes other than those due to increased articular blood flow. A variety of methods for quantifying synovitis using these radioisotopes have been devised but none have achieved uniform acceptance. It seems that the measurement of the absolute uptake per unit joint area produces the best separation between rheumatoid and normal joints, and this can be used in assessing the efficacy of NSAIDs. Radionuclide scanning of the sacro–iliac joints has been used as a diagnostic tool in the sero-negative arthropathies and in assessing drug therapy. The usefulness of sacro–iliac joint scanning is improved by comparing the peak uptake of each sacro–iliac joint with uptake over the sacrum. Unfortunately, there is some overlap in the sacro–iliac/sacral ratio between normal and abnormal individuals which reduces its usefulness as a diagnostic test, although significant reduction in these ratios can be demonstrated after as little as three-weeks' treatment with NSAIDs.

NSAIDs are known to significantly reduce the heat produced by inflamed joints and this can be measured in a variety of ways. Modern infra-red thermography provides a detailed pattern of the heat emanating from a joint surface which can be displayed on a video screen. However, practical considerations such as the high cost of the equipment and the fact that all measurements must be made in a controlled temperature area have meant that thermography has not been used extensively for assessing the efficacy of NSAIDs. Changes in the thermographic index have been shown to occur with NSAID therapy and these correlate with other clinical measures of disease activity. However, by comparing clinical indices, radioisotope uptake and thermography in the assessment of knee inflammation, it has been shown that differences in the time course of the rate of change occur. Thus, different aspects of the inflammatory response are probably being assessed by each technique.

Slow-acting anti-rheumatic drugs and immuno-suppressive agents

Although SAARDs will alter many of the end points mentioned previously, they have specific effects on a number of laboratory measures of disease activity. Of the laboratory tests most frequently employed to measure disease activity, the ESR is the most commonly used. Concentrations of a number of acute-phase reactants including C-reactive protein, haptoglobin, fibrinogen, and alpha-2 macroglobulin correlate well with disease activity and are good measures of response to gold, chloroquine, D-penicillamine and corticosteroids. Recently, these parameters have been used to demonstrate the efficacy of salazopyrine and captopril in the treatment of rheumatoid arthritis. Concentrations of acute-phase reactants will usually begin to fall within two weeks of commencing SAARDs and may continue to do so for a period of months. Failure of these drugs to rapidly reduce these concentrations may be associated with a lack of clinical response. High concentrations of C-reactive protein are an indication of severe rheumatoid arthritis and patients with high concentrations are more likely to develop erosive disease. Thus, acute-phase reactants are not only useful in assessing the efficacy of SAARDs, but also in determining which patients should be treated early with these drugs.

The essential amino acid L-tryptophan is displaced from serum albumin by D-penicillamine, gold and chloroquine as well as by NSAIDs. However, whereas NSAIDs alter serum tryptophan concentrations immediately, changes following gold or D-penicillamine can take up to two months. Sulphydryl concentrations are, likewise, increased.

Although rheumatoid factor titres are associated with active rheumatoid arthritis they bear little relationship to other parameters of disease activity. Titres of IgM rheumatoid factor usually fall in patients with rheumatoid arthritis treated with SAARDs or immunosuppressive agents, but are not considered reliable measures of patient response to these drugs. Immunoglobulin concentrations fall during treatment with gold, D-penicillamine and other SAARDs, while albumin concentrations increase. Thus, many of these changes are likely to be secondary to an overall effect on disease activity.

Changes in the concentrations of inflammatory proteins within the synovial fluid tend to reflect plasma concentrations and, although serial biopsy of synovial membrane may be useful in the long term, to assess disease activity and the effect of SAARDs, problems of biopsy variability have to be appreciated. The end point of active rheumatoid arthritis is the reduction of cartilage erosion and joint deformity. The suppression of disease activity may reduce the rate at which erosions develop, or perhaps allow them to heal. This is considered by many clinicians to be one of the features of a slow-acting or immunosuppressive anti-rheumatic agents. The problems with using radiological assessment of anti-rheumatic therapy are primarily methodological. Inter- and intra-observer disagreement is high and this must be taken into consideration when radiological assessments are used. In a recent review of anti-rheumatic drug therapy gold and cyclophosphamide were found to retard the radiographic progression of joint destruction and, although it is likely that other SAARDs have similar effects, there are currently no data to support this contention.

Summary

As yet there is no single measure to adequately reflect the changes in joint inflammation produced by analgesics, NSAIDs or specific anti-arthritic drugs. However, by using a number of clinical and laboratory measures, assessments of patient response to therapy and the relative efficacy of treatments can be made.

Further reading

Buchanan, W. W. and Tugwell, P., 1983, Traditional assessments of articular disease. *Clinics in the Rheumatic Diseases*, **9**, 515–529.

Cooper, S. A., 1983, Models for clinical assessment of oral analgesics. *American Journal of Medicine*, supplement, November, pp. 24–29.

Dixon, J. S., 1982, Biochemical and clinical changes in rheumatoid arthritis: their relationship to the action of anti-rheumatoid drugs. *Seminars in Arthritis and Rheumatism*, **12**, 191–207.

Huskisson, E. C., 1974, Simple analgesics for arthritis. *British Medical Journal*, **4**, 196–200.

Iannuzzi, L., Dawson, N., Zein, N. and Kusaner, I., 1983, Does drug therapy slow radiographic deterioration in rheumatoid arthritis? *New England Journal of Medicine*, **309**, 1023–1028.

Liang, M. H., Cullen, K. E. and Larson, M. G., 1983, Measuring function and health status in rheumatic disease clinical trials. *Clinics in the Rheumatic Diseases*, **9**, 531–539.

Littlejohns, D. W., and Vere, D. W., 1981, The clinical assessment of analgesic drugs. *British Journal of Clinical Pharmacology*, **11**, 319–332.

Ritchie, D. M., Boyle, J. A., McInnes, J. M., Jasani, M. E., Dalakos, T. G., Grieveson, P., and Buchanan, W. W., 1968, Clinical studies with an articular index for the assessment of joint tenderness in patients with rheumatoid arthritis. *Quarterly Journal of Medicine New Series*, **37**, 393–406.

Sharp, J. T., 1983, Radiographic evaluation of the course of articular disease. *Clinics in the Rheumatic Diseases*, **9** 541–557.

3. Analgesics

There are three types of analgesic:

1. Non-acidic anti-pyretic *p*-aminophenol derivatives (e.g., paracetamol).
2. Non-steroidal anti-inflammatory, antipyretic acids (e.g., aspirin, indomethacin etc.)
3. Opium alkaloids and their derivatives (e.g., codeine).

Most rheumatologists believe that NSAIDs relieve pain by virtue of their anti-inflammatory effect, and do not consider them 'pure' analgesics. Certainly, drugs such as meperidine and pentazocine have relatively weak analgesic effects in patients with inflammatory joint disease. However, the NSAIDs are analgesic when tested in acute pain models. Some workers have suggested that they are analgesic in low doses and anti-inflammatory in high doses. However, Kantor has made the point that there is probably a continuum between the two pharmacological effects of analgesic and anti-inflammatory action. Some NSAIDs, such as aspirin and ibuprofen, are marketed as 'over-the-counter' analgesics.

In this chapter paracetamol (acetaminophen) and the opium alkaloids and their derivatives will be considered. Surveys of drug-prescribing in patients with rheumatoid arthritis indicate that some 40% of patients regularly take analgesic preparations, mostly in the form of paracetamol. There is controversy in the literature as to whether paracetamol is effective in relieving pain in rheumatoid arthritis, some workers finding that it does and others that it does not. Narcotic analgesics work entirely within the central nervous system, and have no peripheral action. Since they are not infrequently prescribed to rheumatic patients their clinico-pharmacological actions will be discussed.

The physiology of pain

Pain is the predominant concern of patients with rheumatic disease and the relief of pain a major goal of rheumatologists. Over the past decade, much has been learnt about the physiology of pain and this can be summarized as follows:

Noxious stimuli excite free nerve endings in the tissues (figure 3.1). These nerve endings are the peripheral terminations of small diameter, unmyelinated,

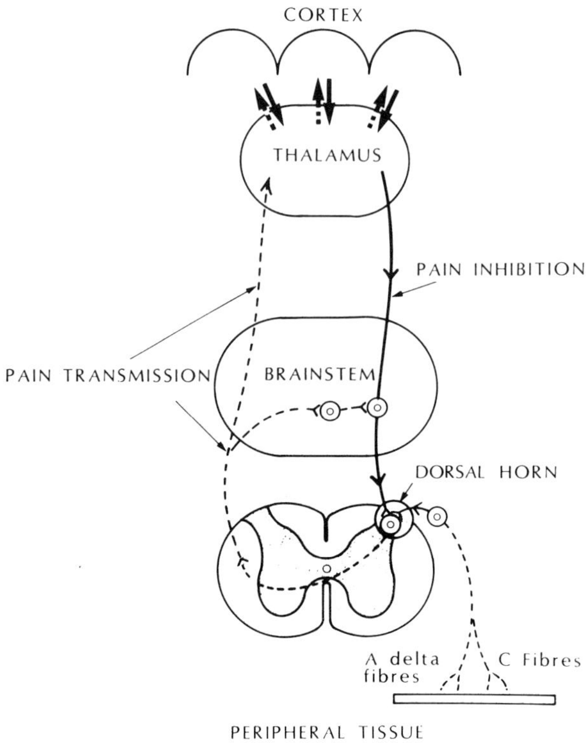

Figure 3.1. Pathways of pain perception.

slow-conducting C fibres. Tissue injury causes the accumulation of chemical mediators which 'fire' the free nerve endings (nociceptors), or, in low concentrations, reduce their threshold to other stimuli, such as heat or pressure. The chemical mediators (algesic) include potassium and hydrogen ions, bradykinin, prostaglandins, histamine and serotonin.

The pain 'message' travels from the free endings through the peripheral nerves to the dorsal horn of the spinal cord, and thence, by many pathways, to thc brainstem, thalamus and cortex. The lateral spinothalamic tract forms one of these pathways and carries signals related to rapidly conducted, well-localized pain from the A delta fibres. It probably mediates acute short-lived pain, whereas the other pathways, many of which originate in the C fibres, carry signals of diffuse and chronic pain.

Recent evidence shows that the impact of a noxious stimulus is modulated in a number of ways so that the pain experienced is not simply a function of the sensory input. The gate-control theory proposes that neural mechanisms in the dorsal horns of the spinal cord act like a gate, increasing and decreasing the flow of nerve impulses travelling up from the peripheral nerves. The dorsal horn of the spinal cord is a complex structure with a multiple array of nerve cells. Some of these neurones, when activated by large fibres not associated with pain, such as light touch, vibration, and pressure, can inhibit the propagation of pain. There is evidence that the sensory input of pain is further modulated at successive synapses throughout its course from the dorsal horn to the brainstem, thalamus and cortex.

The neurones of the dorsal horn and other parts of the central nervous system communicate with each other by means of chemical neurotransmitters, such as enkephalins, serotonin, substance P and noradrenalin. Those neurones which secrete substance P aid the passage of the pain impulse from the peripheral nerve into the spinal cord and brain. Those neurones in the dorsal horn which secrete enkephalins are powerful inhibitors of pain transmission. There are a number of pathways that inhibit pain. They originate in the higher centres of the brain and descend to the enkephalin-secreting neurones of the dorsal horn. These carry signals which stimulate the encephalin-secreting cells in the brainstem, and may partly explain stress-induced analgesia.

Endogenous opioids

The methionine (met) and leucine (leu) enkephalins were first identified in 1975. Endogenous opioids are for the most part peptides, although recently non-peptide endogenous opioids have been described. The term endorphin, coined from 'endogenous morphine,' is used to describe them. The enkephalins, of which there are now seven, are a subclass of these endorphins, and others include alpha-, beta- and gamma-endorphins, and anodynin. Endorphins can be measured by bioassay, radioreceptor, and radio-immune techniques.

Beta-endorphin is present in the anterior and intermediate lobes of the pituitary and in different parts of the brain, but especially in the hypothalamus. It can be detected in both blood and cerebrospinal fluid, and there is now good evidence that the beta-endorphin found in the brain, originates in the neurones of the hypothalamus. The enkephalins are found in the posterior lobe of the pituitary and in different areas of the brain. Both beta-endorphin and the enkephalins are also found in tissues outside the central nervous system, particularly in the cells of the gastro-intestinal tract.

Beta-endorphin has been studied in various clinical states. Elevated concentrations, in both blood and CSF, have been recorded in heroin addicts and in subjects undergoing strenuous physical exercise, while surgical stress and morphine have been noted to cause an increase in blood concentration only. Cushing's syndrome has been associated with decreased levels in the CSF, and dexamethasone results in a fall in blood concentration.

At the present time the natural endorphins have no clinical use because of their enzymatic instability and poor passage across the blood–brain barrier.

However, it is interesting that enzyme inhibitors potentiate their analgesic activity, while naloxone blocks it. Many analogues have been synthesized in an effort to block enzymatic degradation, and are undergoing trials in humans. Further advances are expected in the near future.

Paracetamol (acetaminophen)

Paracetamol (acetaminophen), 4-acetamidophenol (figure 3.2), was first described as an analgesic and anti-pyretic at the end of the last century. In the late 1940s, it was confirmed to be the active metabolite of acetanilide and phenacetin, both of which have now been discarded because of their toxic effects.

Chemistry

The anti-pyretic activity of paracetamol resides in its amino-benzene structure, while the addition of the acetyl group reduces its toxicity.

Pharmacology

Paracetamol has similar anti-pyretic analgesic activity to aspirin, but is a weak inhibitor of prostaglandin synthesis, and therefore has weak anti-inflammatory activity. There is some evidence to suggest that paracetamol blocks prostaglandin synthetase in the central nervous system and this may account for its anti-pyretic properties.

Pharmacokinetics

Paracetamol is rapidly and almost completely absorbed from the gastro-intestinal tract after oral administration. The rate is influenced by the rate of gastric emptying, since paracetamol is absorbed mainly from the small intestine. Peak concentrations are usually achieved within 30 to 90 minutes, but occasionally may take up to 180 minutes.

The presence of food in the stomach delays gastric emptying and the consequent absorption of paracetamol. Drugs which delay gastric emptying, such

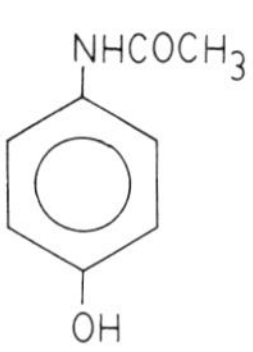

Figure 3.2. Paracetamol (acetaminophen).

as propantheline and meperidine hydrochloride, cause a delay in absorption too: drugs which promote gastric emptying, such as metoclopramide, have the opposite effect. Alterations in gastric pH, as in achlorhydria, have no appreciable effect on paracetamol absorption. Patients who ingest paracetamol at night, immediately before sleeping, excrete less than when they take the same dose in the morning.

Differences have been observed in the absorption characteristics of different oral preparations. Thus, paracetamol is absorbed faster as an effervescent formulation or aqueous suspension than as a compressed tablet. Paracetamol–sorbitol formulations produce higher blood concentrations of paracetamol than ordinary paracetamol tablets. Why sorbitol improves paracetamol absorption is unknown, but this effect could be due to the rapid dissolution of combined tablets or an increase in gastric peristalsis. Paracetamol does not appear to be as well absorbed from suppositories as from tablets.

Paracetamol is distributed evenly throughout the body fluids. The binding of the drug to plasma proteins varies with dose, up to 50% being bound at the plasma concentrations seen in acute intoxication. Protein binding is slightly higher in neonates than in adults. The concentration of paracetamol in the CSF is approximately half that of plasma, and because it is a non-ionized, lipid-soluble compound it readily penetrates brain tissue. Paracetamol penetrates breast milk slowly, attaining much lower concentrations than in plasma, and when taken by a nursing mother in therapeutic doses, poses no risk to the infant.

The drug is metabolized in the liver and the inactive metabolic products are excreted by the kidney. The renal clearance of unchanged paracetamol accounts for 2% of the total amount excreted in the urine. With therapeutic doses, approximately 55% can be recovered, in the urine, as a glucuronide conjugate, 25% as a sulphate conjugate, 7% as a catechol derivative, and a further 7% as cysteine and mercapturic acid conjugates (figure 3.2). The latter pathway is catalysed by the cytochrome P-450 mixed-function-oxidase system, which is thought to form an intermediate compound, N-acetyl-*p*-benzoquinoneimine. This reactive, intermediate metabolite is normally inactivated immediately by liver glutathione, and the cysteine and mercapturic acid conjugates produced excreted in the urine.

With therapeutic doses of paracetamol (i.e. 4 g/day, or less, in an adult), very little of this reactive intermediate is produced, and sufficient hepatic glutathione is present to conjugate with it. However, like all enzymes, those which metabolize paracetamol to the glucuronide and sulphate conjugates display kinetics of the Michaelis–Menten type. Thus, at high concentrations the enzyme system becomes saturated, changing from a first-order to a zero-order rate; as a consequence, the half-life of elimination of the drug increases with the dose. This phenomenon can be seen at high therapeutic and toxic doses, and in this regard paracetamol is similar to the salicylates.

After a single 3 g dose of paracetamol, the sulphate pathway becomes saturated, and doses higher than this saturate the glucuronide pathway. Thus with toxic doses of paracetamol the major pathway of metabolism occurs through the P-450 mixed-function-oxidase system. When the rate of production of the toxic intermediate formed by this system exceeds glutathione production by the liver, the compound binds covalently to hepatocyte macromolecules, causing cell death. However, the depletion of glutathione alone, in the absence of this toxic intermediate, does not cause necrosis.

Paracetamol metabolism takes place exclusively in the liver. In anephric patients there is no formation of sulphate, glucuronide or other metabolites.

It has been known for some time that alcoholics, epileptics, and those with severe liver disease are susceptible to the hepatotoxic effects of paracetamol. Alcohol, phenytoin, phenobarbitone, and rifampicin cause enzyme induction of cytochrome P-450, leading to increased activity of the enzyme and consequent depletion of glutathione. A low protein diet or the administration of dimethyl malate depletes glutathione stores also, and potentiates paracetamol hepatotoxicity. Patients with severe liver damage have difficulty in metabolizing paracetamol, but, in recommended therapeutic dosage, paracetamol appears quite safe in those with well compensated liver disease.

The biological half-life of paracetamol is of the order of two hours in healthy adult subjects. This is somewhat longer in neonates, who have a reduced capacity to produce glucuronide conjugates, but have more rapid sulphate formation. The relatively low incidence of hepatic toxicity in children who have received an overdose of paracetamol may be due to their having less cytochrome P-450 oxidase activity than adults. In elderly patients, there is conflicting evidence as to whether the elimination half-life of the drug is prolonged. However, a recent study has shown that an alteration of dosage on the basis of pharmacokinetic data is not justified. Large doses of vitamin C (3 g or more) cause prolongation of the biological half-life of paracetamol by competing for the sulphate used in its metabolism (figure 3.3).

Renal clearance of paracetamol is related to the rate of urinary flow, but not to urinary pH. However, the rate of clearance of the conjugates is affected neither by renal flow nor urinary pH. The excretory process of paracetamol involves glomerular filtration and passive re-absorption throughout the entire length of the nephron. Both sulphate and glucuronide conjugates undergo glomerular filtration: at low plasma concentrations both are secreted by active transport while at higher concentrations both are actively re-absorbed. Impairment of renal function leads to a delay in the excretion of paracetamol and its metabolites; there is a significant correlation between 24-hour creatinine clearance and the clearance of free and bound paracetamol.

In contrast to aspirin and phenacetin, acute ingestion of paracetamol causes only a slight increase in renal-tubular-cell excretion. In patients with rheumatoid arthritis no relationship between paracetamol consumption and serum-creatinine concentration, creatinine clearance, urinary-concentrating

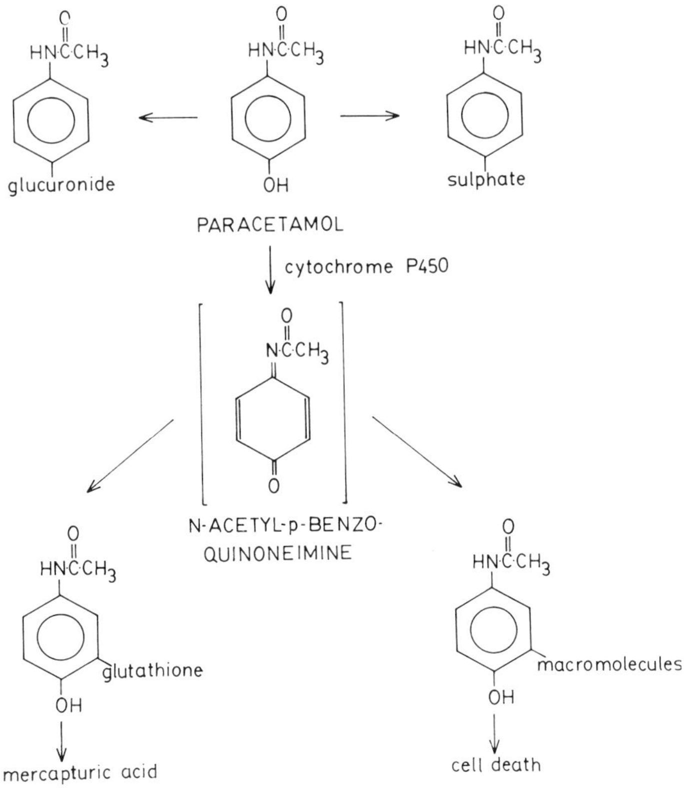

Figure 3.3. Paracetamol metabolism.

capacity, titratable acidity or ammonium excretion has been found. Nor has any deterioration been observed in patients with rheumatoid arthritis treated chronically with therapeutic doses of paracetamol (4 g/day). In overdosage, paracetamol may cause acute tubular necrosis, which is often, but not always, associated with acute hepatic failure. This does not appear to be caused by the so-called hepato–renal syndrome, but by direct nephrotoxicity, and is potentiated by the depletion of glutathione.

Thus, despite its extensive use, there is little evidence that paracetamol alone, in therapeutic doses, causes renal damage. Nevertheless, since paracetamol is a major metabolite of phenacetin it is important that continued critical appraisal of its long-term use be made, especially in relation to renal function.

Paracetamol potentiates the effect of vasopressin *in vitro*. In patients with diabetes insipidus, doses of between 1 and 2.5 g produce an increase in urine osmolarity and a fall in urine flow rate and water clearance.

Table 3.1. Clinically relevant drug interactions of paracetamol.

Drug	**Clinical effect**	**Explanation**
Food	Delays absorption	Slows gastric-emptying time. Some evidence that pectin in carbohydrates depresses rate of absorption
Propantheline Meperidine hydrochloride	Delays absorption	Slows gastric emptying time
Metoclopramide	Accelerates absorption	Increases gastric-emptying time
Ethyl alcohol Phenobarbitone Phenytoin Rifampicin	Predisposes to hepatic damage	Induces cytochrome P450 enzyme, resulting in depletion of glutathione

Drug interactions

In man, the concurrent administration of codeine and caffeine does not significantly alter the metabolism of paracetamol. The important interactions and their mechanisms are summarized in table 3.1. There is no significant interaction between paracetamol and anticoagulants, and cimetidine has been shown to have no effect on the metabolism of paracetamol.

Toxicity

Paracetamol rarely causes adverse reactions at recommended therapeutic doses. Hypersensitivity is extremely rare, and responds rapidly to drug withdrawal. Reversible haematological abnormalities have been described, but are extremely rare.

Hepatic damage occurs with drug overdose only. Patients who have developed hepatic damage with long-term use have either used doses higher than recommended, have had some predisposing cause, such as chronic alcoholism, or have taken drugs likely to cause enzyme induction in the liver e.g. phenytoin and phenobarbitone. The pathogenesis of liver damage is due to the depletion of hepatic glutathione, which normally inactivates the toxic intermediate, N-acetyl-*p*-benzoquinoneimine. This intermediate metabolite binds to hepatocytes causing cell death. The major pathological feature of this form of hepatic damage is centri-zonal necrosis.

There appears to be no hepatic damage following the ingestion of less than 125 mg/kg, but the incidence and severity increase significantly with doses of 250 mg/kg or more. Plasma concentrations provide useful indicators of potential liver damage: concentrations exceeding 300 μg/ml four hours after ingestion are consistently associated with liver damage while those below

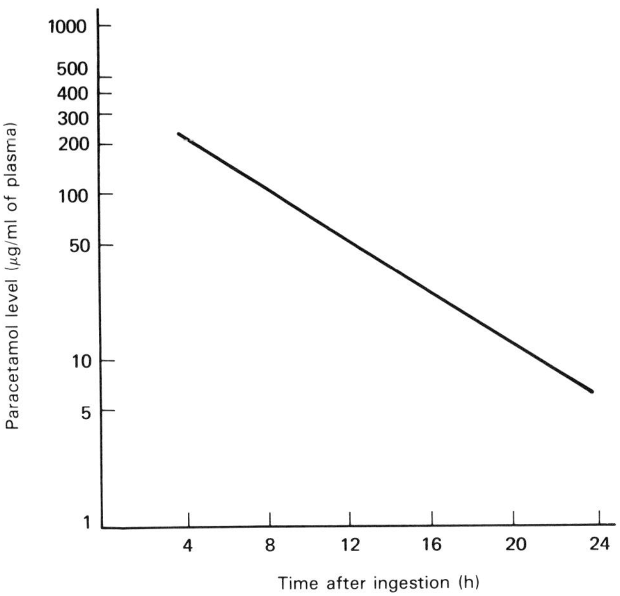

Figure 3.4. A semi-logarithmic plot of plasma paracetamol concentration versus time. The area above the line indicates probable hepatotoxic reaction and that below the line, no hepatotoxic reaction. (Published by permission of Dr. Barry H. Rumack and the Editor of *Archives of Internal Medicine*).

120 μg/ml are not. It should be noted that these plasma concentrations far exceed the peak therapeutic level of 15 μg/ml after a single dose of 1 g.

Nomograms have been published for assessing the potential toxicity of paracetamol overdosage (figure 3.4). Substances which serve as precursors of cysteine (methionine and acetylcysteine) and thus of glutathione, have been used as antidotes. In addition, nucleophils such as mercaptamine which combine with the toxic metabolite have been sought. However, mercaptamine may also inhibit the formation of the toxic metabolite.

Codeine

Codeine (figure 3.5) is a natural opium alkaloid in which the phenolic hydroxyl group of morphine is replaced by a methoxyl group. The drug was discovered just over 150 years ago, and recognized as a methyl ether of morphine in 1882. The degree to which codeine's analgesic effect is mediated by biotransformation to morphine is uncertain, but there is evidence that codeine is not entirely a pro-drug. In clinical practice codeine is considered 'mild' when administered orally, and, with the exception of aspirin, it is the most widely used analgesic. Controlled clinical trials have shown that 60 or 65 mg of codeine is significantly superior to placebo as an analgesic, and some but not all trials have even

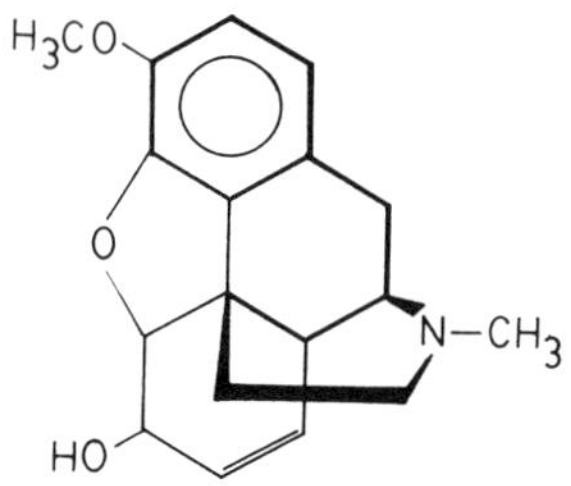

Figure 3.5. Codeine.

shown that half this dose, when given orally, is superior to placebo. Codeine is ten times as effective as aspirin as an analgesic on a weight basis. Thus, codeine, in doses of 60 to 65 mg, and aspirin, in doses of 600 to 650 mg, are equipotent. In some studies, codeine was found to be superior to propoxyphene in equivalent milligram doses, but other studies have shown the two drugs to be equally effective.

Pharmacology and pharmacokinetics

The opioids are readily absorbed from the gastro-intestinal tract, and codeine is no exception. Indeed, in contrast to morphine, codeine is approximately two thirds as effective orally as parenterally, both as an analgesic and a respiratory depressant. In one series of experiments the oral/parenteral potency ratio was 0.68 for codeine and 0.17 for morphine. Codeine's greater oral efficacy can be explained by the fact that it is metabolized more thoroughly on its first passage through the liver than morphine. Codeine is also absorbed when administered sublingually, but less well when swallowed. The absorption of codeine after subcutaneous injection is better than that of morphine.

Once absorbed codeine is metabolized extensively in the liver: only a small amount of free codeine is excreted in the urine, the greater part appearing as metabolites. Figure 3.6 illustrates the major metabolic pathways for codeine.

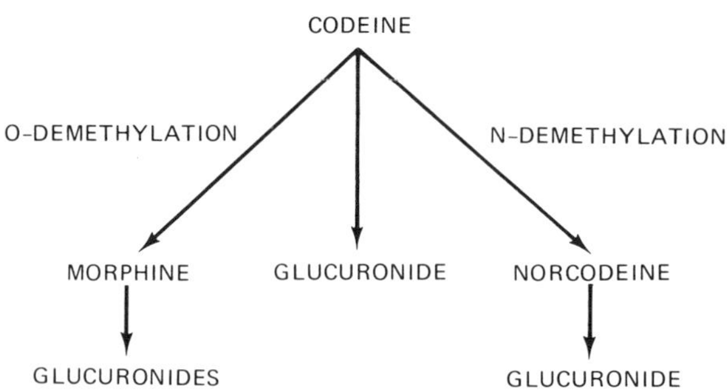

Figure 3.6. Codeine metabolism.

Approximately 10% is demethylated to morphine. Smoking has no effect on metabolism and the plasma half-life, after both oral and parenteral administration, is two to three hours: the corresponding clinical analgesic effect last about four to six hours.

Morphine readily crosses the placental barrier and may cause respiratory depression in the newborn infant. There is no clear evidence that codeine will do the same, but it is suspected. Nevertheless, in view of codeine's greater first-pass metabolism in the liver, it would be likely to cause less respiratory depression in the neonate than morphine. Codeine is weakly basic and highly lipophilic, and is excreted in milk, where it appears in higher concentration than in plasma.

Drug interactions

CNS depression by codeine is augmented by alcohol, sedatives, hypnotics, tranquillizers and other depressants.

Side-effects

Undoubtedly, the most common side-effect of codeine is constipation. Codeine is less sedative and emetic than morphine, but liable to tolerance. Headache, dizziness, lightheadedness, and sweating may occur after codeine administration, but are relatively uncommon. Allergic phenomena occur, but are rare. Since codeine is metabolized in the liver it should be used with caution in patients with severe liver disease. Displacement of the alveolar pCO_2-response curve, in normal subjects, has been demonstrated with as little as a 60 mg oral dose. Thus, codeine, like other opiates, should be used with great caution in patients with decreased respiratory reserve, as in bronchial asthma, emphysema, severe kyphoscoliosis, and morbid obesity. A fall in blood pressure may occur after the parenteral administration of codeine, and, therefore, it should be avoided in patients with reduced blood volume, as after haemorrhage. Likewise, it should be avoided in patients with head injury, as the effects of respiratory depressant are exaggerated with increased intracranial pressure, and in patients with prostatic hypertrophy, since it is well known that morphine may precipitate acute urinary retention. One of the major limitations to the use of opioids is the development of tolerance and physical dependence. Addiction to codeine, however, is extremely rare, and the drug can be used safely in recommended therapeutic doses, for long periods, without any side-effects other than constipation.

Dihydrocodeine

Dihydrocodeine (figure 3.7) is commonly used for mild to moderate pain, including rheumatic pain. The metabolism of the drug has not been established,

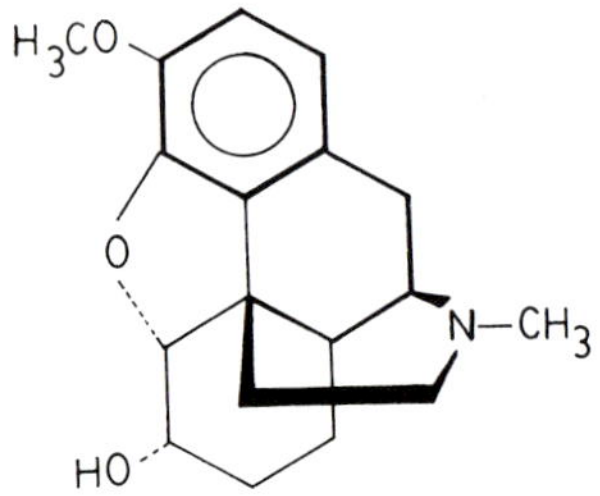

Figure 3.7. Dihydrocodeine.

but it probably undergoes a biotransformation similar to that of codeine, with dihydrocodeine-6-glucuronide as the major metabolite. After an oral dose, the peak plasma concentrations are achieved within about one-and-a-half hours, the absorption rate being constant and independent of the dose. The bioavailability of dihydrocodeine is approximately 20%; whether this is due to poor gastro-intestinal absorption or substantial pre-systemic metabolism within the intestinal wall or liver is not known. Clearance of dihydrocodeine is not dose-dependent and its duration of action is between four and six hours.

The unwanted effects of dihydrocodeine are similar to those of morphine, but less pronounced. Pre-existing respiratory depression is a definite contra-indication, as is hypersensitivity to codeine. Caution in prescribing the drug to patients with renal failure is necessary, probably because uraemia leads to a reduction of protein-binding, resulting in higher free concentrations and side-effects. Alcohol, sedatives, hypnotics, and tranquillizers cause increased CNS depression when given concurrently with dihydrocodeine. Long-term use by susceptible individuals may lead to habituation. Naloxone is useful in the treatment of overdose.

Oxycodone

Oxycodone (dihydrohydroxycodeinone) (figure 3.8) is a semi-synthetic analogue of morphine, which can be administered as the hydrochloride, either

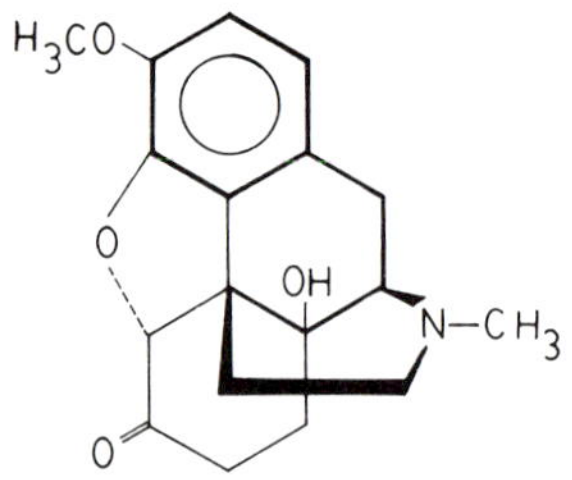

Figure 3.8. Oxycodone.

orally or by injection. Oxycodone pectinate is available as rectal tablets (about 30 mg being clinically equivalent to 20 mg morphine hydrochloride, given orally, or 6 to 7 mg given by subcutaneous or intra-muscular injection).

There is comparatively little data on the pharmacokinetics of oxycodone, though the drug is rapidly absorbed after oral administration and its duration of action is similar to that of morphine, lasting four to six hours.

Oxycodone differs from morphine in its quantitative, but not qualitative characteristics. Thus, oxycodone may cause gastro-intestinal side-effects, such as nausea, vomiting and constipation, and CNS effects, including light-headedness, dizziness, sedation, euphoria and dysphoria. Patients should be cautioned that their mental and physical alertness may be impaired, and the drug should be used with caution in the elderly and debilitated. Dependence may occur with long-term use. Oxycodone should be avoided, if possible, in patients with cardiac and respiratory depression and those with hepatic and renal failure. Respiratory depression may occur in the newborn. Occasionally, patients develop pruritus.

Drug interactions include the potentiation of CNS depression with alcohol, sedatives, hypnotics and other depressants.

Pentazocine

Pentazocine (figure 3.9) is a narcotic analgesic which is approximately one third as potent as morphine when given intramuscularly. It has the advantage over morphine in that it is active when orally administered. Another advantage is that it is significantly less addictive. Pentazocine relieves pain, but has no place in the management of arthritic disorders. However, it is not infrequently used by family doctors to relieve severe joint pain and, therefore, it is important that clinical rheumatologists have knowledge of the drug and its effects.

The peak plasma concentration occurs 3 hours after oral administration and 15 minutes to 1 hour after parenteral administration.

First-pass metabolism in the liver is extensive and less than 20% of pentazocine enters the systemic circulation. For this reason the oral dose is five times less effective than the same dose given parenterally. However, the oral to

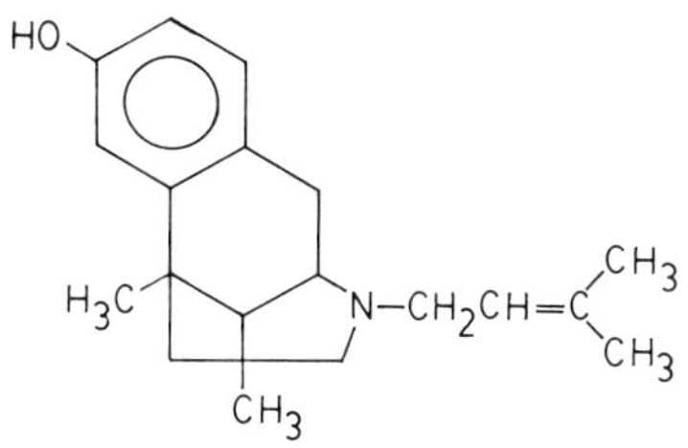

Figure 3.9. Pentazocine.

parenteral efficacy ratio is better for pentazocine than for most of the narcotic analgesics. The drug is extensively metabolized in the liver, but the rate of metabolism varies between individuals and this may account for the variability in analgesic response. The plasma half-life is two to three hours.

Approximately 50% of the drug is bound to plasma proteins, and 33% is found in the red blood cells. The latter may be due to the fact that the drug is highly lipid soluble.

Only a small amount of free pentazocine is excreted in the urine, most of the drug being metabolized in the liver. Pentazocine does not possess the anti-diuretic activity characteristic of morphine, but urine retention may occur. Thus, the drug should be used cautiously in patients with renal impairment.

The analgesic activity of pentazocine is due mainly to the L-isomer. The onset of analgesia is 15 to 20 minutes after intramuscular doses and 2 to 3 minutes following intravenous doses. The effect usually lasts about three hours.

Side-effects

The most common side-effects are sedation, dizziness or lightheadedness, sweating, and nausea. Vomiting is less frequent than with morphine. The respiratory depressant properties of pentazocine, like morphine, are almost confined to the L-isomer and are antagonized by naloxone. Pentazocine does not appear to have depressant effects on cardiac output and is less likely to produce hypotension than morphine. No haematological, renal or hepatic disturbances have been reported with the use of pentazocine, but since the drug is extensively metabolized in the liver, it should be used cautiously in patients with hepatic impairment.

Pentazocine is not euphorogenic and because of this it is less likely to produce addiction than morphine. Rarely, naloxone-like psychiatric effects including strange thoughts and hallucinations have been reported.

Propoxyphene

Propoxyphene (figure 3.10) is a mild analgesic which is structurally related to the narcotic analgesic methadone. The analgesic activity is due to the D-isomer, whereas L-propoxyphene has some anti-tussive activity. Despite the widespread use of propoxyphene, there have been relatively few controlled therapeutic trials to testify to its efficacy. In other trials the drug has been found to be no better than placebo as an analgesic. Furthermore, there is little evidence that combinations of propoxyphene with other analgesics are superior to one analgesic alone. Aspirin and paracetamol appear to be just as effective when given alone as when administered with propoxyphene. Propoxyphene binds to opioid receptors and produces an analgesia similar to that of codeine and other opioids. It has no anti-pyretic or anti-inflammatory effects.

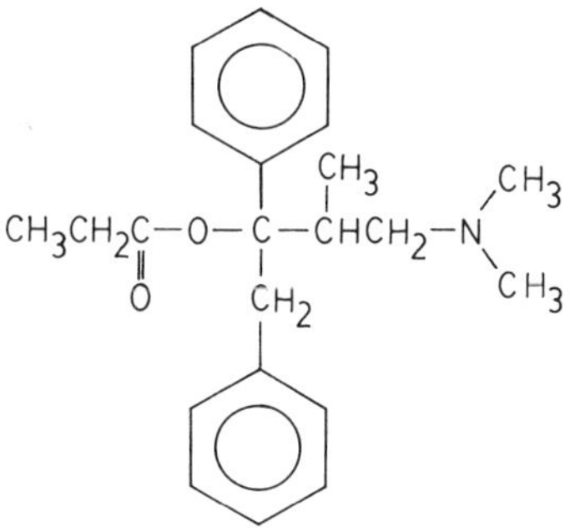

Fig. 3.10. Propoxyphene.

Propoxyphene is rapidly absorbed from the gastro-intestinal tract after oral administration, peak plasma concentrations appearing within one to two hours. The dosage formulation appears to have little effect on absorption, although the water insoluble napsylate salt would seem to have a slower absorption than the hydrochloride.

Propoxyphene has a relatively low systemic availability after oral ingestion, due to its metabolism on first pass through the liver. After a dose of 65 mg, about 20% reaches the systemic circulation unaltered. The major route of metabolism is N-demethylation to norpropoxyphene, which is slowly excreted in the urine. There is considerable variation between individuals in terms of the plasma concentration of propoxyphene, and metabolism is more rapid in smokers. The mean plasma half-life, following oral administration, is approximately 12 hours, and with repeated 6 hourly oral doses a steady state is reached in 1 to 2 days.

Caffeine

For many years caffeine (figure 3.11) has been an ingredient of analgesic mixtures containing aspirin, phenacetin, paracetamol, propoxyphene and salicylamide. Their widespread use by millions of patients attests to their appeal, and could be taken to prove efficacy. However, in 1977 *The Food and Drug Administration Advisory Review Panel on Over-the Counter Internal*

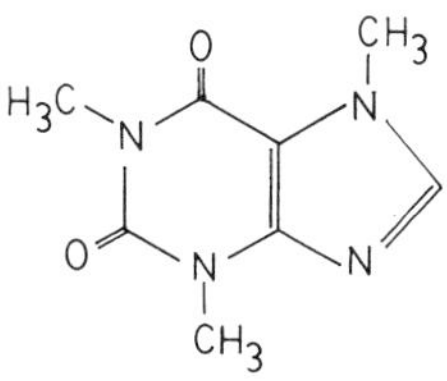

Figure 3.11. Caffeine.

Analgesics, Anti-Pyretic and Anti-Rheumatic Products in the USA concluded that, "there are insufficient data to demonstrate any additional contribution of caffeine" to the action of these analgesic mixtures. This view, as shared by many authoritative medical texts, journal articles, and advisory letters, indicated that both the public and medical profession had been wrong in assuming caffeine to be an adjuvant. Recently, Laska and his colleagues re-analysed the 30 randomized, controlled trials, involving more than 10 000 patients, carried out over the past 20 years, to assess whether caffeine was an analgesic adjuvant or not. The overall pooled relative potency estimate was 1.41, with 95% confidence limits or 1.23 to 1.63, that is, to obtain the same analgesic response without caffeine, would require a dose that is approximately 40% greater. Thus, caffeine's contribution to the efficacy of over-the-counter and prescription analgesic combinations is real, but modest. The minimum effective dose of caffeine appears to be 65 mg. The optimal dose has not been determined, but empirically 100 to 200 mg would seem appropriate.

Caffeine has been shown to be effective in relieving headache. Whether this effect is due to an analgesic action or to its effect on cerebral blood flow and vascular tone is not known. Caffeine may simply enhance the response to an analgesic by altering the mood, providing a sense of 'well-being'. The pharmacological effects of caffeine are extremely complex and include the translocation of intercellular calcium, the accumulation of cyclic nucleotides (particularly cyclic AMP), blocking adenosine receptors, potentiation of inhibitors of prostaglandin synthesis, reducing catecholamine uptake in non-neural tissue, and inhibition of the release of histamine from mast cells. Further research is required to determine whether any of these pharmacological actions modify pain.

Caffeine, like other methylxanthines, is readily absorbed after oral, parenteral or rectal administration. Maximum concentrations in plasma occur within one hour of oral administration in the absence of food. It is eliminated by metabolism in the liver, 1% only being recovered in the urine unchanged. The half-life of caffeine in plasma is of the order of about three-and-a-half hours in man. Caffeine is distributed into all body compartments, and crosses the placenta. This latter fact is of importance since the half-life of caffeine in premature infants is significantly prolonged, being of the order of 36 to 144 hours. The volume of distribution in the adult is of the order of 400 to 550 ml/kg. Less than 50% of caffeine is bound to plasma proteins, which may account for its ready penetration of brain and CSF, as may its lipid solubility.

The principal metabolites of caffeine recovered in the urine are L-methyluric acid and L-methylxanthine.

Side-effects

Caffeine may cause nervousness, insomnia, headache, nausea and vomiting, palpitation, vertigo, muscle tremor, sensory disturbances, and excessive diuresis in sensitive patients. In rheumatic patients with these symptoms it is prudent to check whether they are having analgesic mixtures containing caffeine. In large doses caffeine may cause gastric irritation.

Further reading

Brooks, P. M., Dougan, M. A., Mugford, S. and Meffin, E., 1982, Comparative effectiveness of five analgesics in patients with rheumatoid arthritis. *Journal of Rheumatology*, **9**, 723–726.

Cooper, S. A., 1983, Models for clinical assessment of oral analgesics. *American Journal of Medicine*, Supplement, pp 24–29.

Huskisson, E. C., 1974, Simple analgesics for arthritis. *British Medical Journal*, **4**, 196–200.

Kantor, T. G., 1980, Analgesics for arthritis. *Clinics in the Rheumatic Diseases*, **6**, 525–531.

Koch-Weser, J., 1976, Acetaminophen, *New England Journal of Medicine*, **295**, 1297–1300.

Laska, E. M., Sunshine, A., Mueller, F., Elvers, W. B., Siegel, C. and Rubin, A., 1984, Caffeine as an analgesic adjuvant. *Journal of the American Medical Association*, **251**, 1711–1718.

Lee, P., Watson, M., Webb, J., Anderson, J., and Buchanan, W., 1975, Therapeutic effectiveness of paracetamol in rheumatoid arthritis. *International Journal of Clinical Pharmacology*, **11**, 68–75.

Melzak, R. and Wall, P. D., 1965, Pain mechanisms: a new theory. *Science*, **150**, 971–979.

Moertel, C. G., Ahmann, D. L., Taylor, W. F. and Schwartau, N., 1972, A comparative evaluation of marketed analgesic drugs. *New England Journal of Medicine*, **286**, 813–815.

Nuki, G., Downie, W. W., Dick, W. C., Whaley, K. *et al.*, 1973, Clinical trial of pentazocine in rheumatoid arthritis. *Annals of the Rheumatic Diseases*, **32**, 436–443.

Rosen Bloom, D., Brooks, P. M., Bellamy, N. and Buchanan, W. W., 1984, *Clinical Trials in the Rheumatic Diseases—a Selected Critical Review*. Praeger, New York.

4. Salicylates

Salicylates, in the leaves and barks of certain trees, have been used for medicinal purposes since ancient times. Hippocrates, Galen and a number of early Greek and Roman herbalists used extracts of bark for pain relief and anti-pyresis. In 1763, the Reverend Edward Stone reported the use of willow bark as an anti-pyretic to the Royal Philosophical Society in London and created an upsurge in interest in bark preparations. Salicylic acid was extracted by a number of European chemists, in the 1800s and Felix Hofmann, a chemist with the Bayer Pharmaceutical Company, developed a commercial method for synthesizing aspirin in 1893. In the treatment of pain and inflammation salicylates still play a major role as the drugs of first choice, although their place has been challenged by some of the newer NSAIDs.

Chemistry

Salicylic acid is the *o*-isomer of hydroxybenzoic acid and aspirin is the common name for its acetate ester (acetylsalicylic acid) (figure 4.1). Both these compounds are relatively insoluble in water, their sodium salts being more soluble.

The solubilities of salicylic acid and aspirin are dependent of a number of physico-chemical properties, including the ionization, the pH of the solution and the formulation of the preparation. Aspirin is relatively unstable, even in the powder form, as it is hydrolysed to salicylic acid and acetic acid in moist air. Thus, care must be taken in the preparation, and storage of solutions,

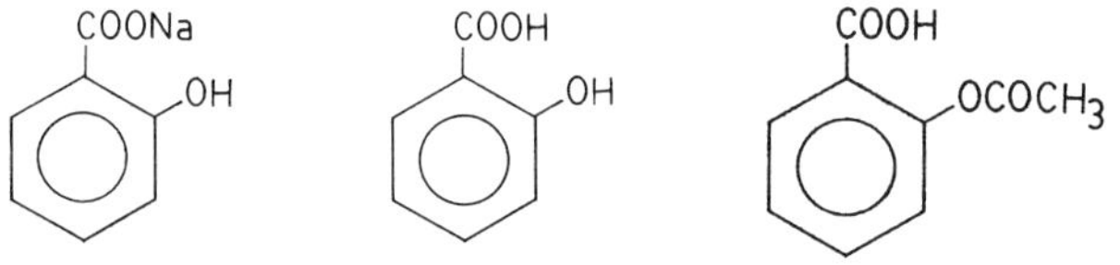

Figure 4.1. Sodium salicylate, salicylic acid and acetylsalicylic acid.

since a freshly prepared solution of aspirin at pH 7.4, stored at 17°C, can be expected to exhibit a 10% hydrolysis to salicylic acid in 24 hours.

Pharmacology

Both salicylic acid and aspirin have a variety of effects *in vitro* and *in vivo*, as shown in table 4.1. One of their principal mechanisms of action is on prostaglandin synthesis and since this was demonstrated in the early 1970s, aspirin has become widely used as a pharmacological tool, not only for modifying inflammation, but also for inhibiting platelet adhesiveness and a variety of other events. This has led to its extensive use, not only in the treatment of inflammation, but also in the prophylaxis of coronary-artery disease, arterial thrombosis and cerebrovascular disorders.

Table 4.1. Mechanism of action of salicylic acid and acetylsalicylic acid.

Effect on	**Salicylic acid**	**Acetylsalicylic acid**
Prostaglandin synthetase	Inhibition weak-reversible	Inhibition strong-irreversible
Lipoxygenase	No effect on HPETE production, but inhibits conversion to HETE	
Lysosomal membranes	Variable effects *in vitro* possibly with stabilization	
Kinin production	Inhibits	Inhibits
Effect of glycolysis and oxidative phosphorylation	Inhibits in supra-physiological concentration, some reversibility *in vitro*	
Effect on free fatty acid	Reduce free fatty acids only in man	
c-AMP concentrations	Reduce c-AMP concentration possibly via prostaglandin inhibition	
Glycosaminoglycan	Decreases glycosaminoglycan production from a variety of cartilage species? c-AMP dependent	
Fibrinolytic activity	Increases *in vitro* and *in vivo*	
Vitamin K-independent coagulation factors	Inhibits production *in vitro* and *in vivo*	
Lymphocyte transformation	*In-vitro* and *in vivo* transformation reduced	
Neutrophil and macrophage production	Inhibition of O_2 production *in vitro* and *in vivo*	
Displaces proteins/drugs from binding sites	Reversible	Irreversible

Although it is relatively easy to separate the effects of aspirin and salicylic acid *in vitro*, it is more difficult to do so *in vivo*. It is also important to appreciate that different concentrations of both drugs have widely differing effects on enzyme systems.

The uncoupling of oxidative phosphorylation by aspirin or salicylic acid can be shown *in vitro* and, although this results in the inhibition of many ATP-dependent reactions, it is unlikely to produce major effects *in vivo* at the plasma concentrations normally achieved. Salicylic acid reduces the plasma concentration of free fatty acids by inhibiting their mobilization from adipose tissue and this appears to result in a secondary increase in insulin concentration.

Salicylates affect the function of enzyme systems *in vitro* and *in vivo*. Some of the enzyme systems shown to be inhibited *in vitro*, by high concentrations of these drugs, include the dehydrogenases involved in oxidative phosphorylation, decarboxylases, amino-tranferases, amino-acyl RNA synthetases, nucleic-acid polymerases and sialyl-tranferases.

The concentration of cAMP in cells is normally elevated by prostaglandin metabolites. Aspirin decreases the cAMP concentration in lymphocytes and inhibits their response to isoprenaline or prostaglandin. Salicylic acid affects cyclic nucleotide concentration also, indicating that its overall effect on the body is not mediated by the inhibition of cyclo-oxygenase alone. In a number of animal species, the production of glycosaminoglycan in the articular cartilage is inhibited by salicylic acid, possibly through its interference with cAMP formation.

Aspirin and salicylic acid have a variety of affects on blood clotting in addition to their effect on platelet cyclo-oxygenase. Both compounds increase the fibrinolytic activity of whole blood and this results in an enhanced euglobulin-lysis time. Vitamin-K-dependent coagulation factors, including prothrombin synthesis, are inhibited by salicylic acid though little effect on bleeding time is observed.

Studies *in vitro* have shown that aspirin binds reversibly to peripheral lymphocytes and inhibits their response to a variety of mitogens. As arachidonic metabolites play a significant role in lymphocyte function, it is obvious that some of the effects of salicylic acid and aspirin will be mediated through this mechanism. In animals models, and *in vitro*, salicylates interfere with the migration of PMNs and macrophages.

High doses of salicylates can cause a variety of toxic effects on the central nervous and respiratory systems and alter the electrolyte and acid–base balance. However, the biochemical mechanisms for many of these effects are unknown. Patients suffering from CNS toxicity present with confusion, dizziness, psychosis or coma; with tinnitus and hearing loss being quite common and related to the plasma concentration of salicylate. Nausea and vomiting occur and may be due to a direct effect on the medulla or as a consequence of local gastric irritation. With therapeutic concentrations of salicylate definite changes in acid–base balance and electrolyte pattern are seen. As a consequence of the salicylate-induced uncoupling of oxidative phosphorylation, both CO_2 production and oxygen consumption increase, respiration is stimulated and a mild respiratory alkalosis occurs. In compensation, the renal excretion of bicarbonate, sodium and potassium is increased and the blood pH returns towards normal. Further changes in electrolyte and acid–base balance occur only if high doses are ingested. In this situation a metabolic acidosis occurs, with subsequent respiratory depression and respiratory acidosis. The consequent loss of sodium, potassium and water results in dehydration.

Salicylates have been shown to cause transient changes in creatinine clearance, renal blood flow and renal tubular-cell excretion in normal people and patients with rheumatoid arthritis. Many of these effects may be mediated by prostaglandins, but their relevance to patients on chronic therapy is unclear. Renin activity, in the plasma, is suppressed by salicylates and blood pressure may be altered. Thus, care should be taken in patients with compromised renal function when prescribing large doses. Salicylates affect uric acid excretion, decreasing urate excretion at low doses (1.5 g/day or less). At doses in excess of 3.5 g/day, uricosuria is induced lowering the concentration of urate in the plasma.

Pharmacokinetics

Aspirin has a plasma half-life of approximately 15 to 20 minutes and is converted to salicylic acid. This hydrolysis is induced by non-specific esterases. During absorption, esterase activity in the gastro-intestinal mucosa contributes significantly. This activity is highest in the cells of the gastric fundus, but may vary considerably with age, sex and disease.

Rapid absorption of salicylates occurs by passive diffusion of non-ionized lipophilic molecules in the stomach. In the neutral environment of the gastric mucosa, these may become ionized, and accumulate. This eventually results in the retrograde diffusion of hydrogen ions and the consequent disruption of the gastric-mucosal barrier. Salicylate absorption is determined by the dissolution rate of the tablet. Salicylate salts are generally more soluble than their parent compounds, with the exception of aluminium salts. Buffered aspirin preparations rapidly form aspirin salts as the tablets disintegrate, enhancing absorption. Salicylates are absorbed from the jejunum and small bowel by passive diffusion, but rectal absorption may occur also.

A number of factors influence salicylate absorption, including the rate of tablet disintegration, particle size of the preparation, contents of the stomach, gastric-emptying time, concurrent drug therapy and conditions such as migraine. Owing to this, considerable inter- and intra-individual variation occurs in salicylate absorption. However, the major factor altering the rate of absorption is the drug formulation itself. The most rapid absorption occurs with effervescent tablets. Slower absorption is obtained when enteric-coated or slow-release preparations are used. Although early enteric-coated preparations were associated with poor bioavailability, recent preparations have a salicylic-acid bioavailability in excess of 90%.

Salicylate pharmacokinetics have been studied in various age groups and disease states. Neonates have reduced serum albumin concentrations and impaired conjugating mechanisms and, therefore eliminate salicyluric acid slowly. Changes in protein binding significantly alter the volume of distribution and highlight the importance of using free concentrations of salicylic acid to estimate the risk of toxicity from overdose, particularly in children. The pharmacokinetic parameters are not influenced by febrile states in children.

No significant differences have been found in the absorption of aspirin between the elderly and young adults. Though serum albumin concentrations are often diminished in patients with rheumatoid arthritis and differences may exist in the free fraction, there is no evidence that the protein binding of salicylate is altered. The free fraction of salicylic acid has been shown to be increased in patients with renal failure, but other pharmacokinetic parameters are unchanged. Unbound concentrations are significantly higher in those patients with liver disease owing to a decrease in the binding and clearance of salicylic acid.

The optimal dose of aspirin required to reduce platelet adhesiveness and maintain the production of vascular prostacyclin is unknown. The effect of aspirin on platelet-membrane cyclo-oxygenase is permanent, but new enzyme can be produced in the vessel walls. A significant reduction in platelet aggregation is seen following doses of 160 mg of soluble aspirin and 650 mg of enteric-coated aspirin. Given once-daily, this dose allows prostacyclin production to be maintained in the vessel walls, while still significantly interfering with platelet adhesiveness. Evidence suggests that aspirin is a better analgesic than salicylic acid and, although the analgesia produced is dose-dependent, it does not seem to parallel concentrations of aspirin in the serum. Furthermore, the dose required for anti-pyresis is less than that required for analgesia.

Although the therapeutic range of salicylate concentrations in the plasma is said to be 1–2 mmol/l no formal studies have been carried out to confirm this. However, it is accepted that doses of salicylic acid in excess of 3 g/day are required to suppress clinical manifestations of inflammation in arthritis. The optimum dose of salicylate in any particular patient is that which maximally suppresses the clinical features of inflammation without causing significant side-effects. The side-effects of salicylate, in particular tinnitus, are related to the total concentration of salicylic acid, but tinnitus is not always a useful practical measure of salicylate toxicity, particularly in the elderly. Indeed, as the optimum plasma concentration is only slightly below toxic levels, care must be taken when they are used. It has been suggested that a reduction in the fractional dose of aspirin, (from 5 to 3 doses per day) will reduce the incidence of side-effects such as tinnitus, but computer simulations have shown that changes in these parameters have little effect on steady-state plasma concentrations. Individualization of dose can be achieved by monitoring plasma concentration, but a number of other variables affecting the elimination of salicylic acid cannot be calculated from this data alone. Nomograms have been developed for guidance, but do not take into consideration the significant inter-individual differences in elimination kinetics. Thus, dose adjustments, in individual patients, need to be based on data obtained from monitoring plasma concentration as well as observations of the patient's clinical state.

In theory, steady-state concentrations of salicylic acid, in the therapeutic range throughout a 24-hour period, are necessary for the ideal management of chronic rheumatic disease. In planning dosage, it is reasonable to commence therapy with 60 mg/kg/day for 1 week, obtain a plasma sample 1 to 3 hours after administration and increase the dose to 80 mg/kg/day if the plasma salicylate concentration is below 1.1 mmol/l. Increases in dose must be made cautiously and should be carried out after thorough clinical and pharmacokinetic assessment of the patient. A 12-hour dosing schedule can be employed using an enteric-coated or a sustained-release preparation. To achieve rapid absorption with peak aspirin levels, effervescent formulations are appropriate. The addition of metoclopramide will further enhance absorption and is recommended in conditions, such as migraine, which are associated with reduced gastric emptying.

Protein binding

Once absorbed, salicylate is distributed among the body fluids. Both drugs are partially bound to serum proteins, primarily albumin; salicylic acid to a greater extent than aspirin. They bind to erythrocytes also. Low concentrations of albumin in rheumatoid arthritis can lead to lower serum salicylate concentrations, making salicylate clearance easier and influencing distribution. In this situation, higher concentrations of free salicylate occur in the plasma. The binding of salicylate to albumin is thought to occur at two primary and a number of secondary sites. At normal therapeutic concentrations (1.1 to 2.2 mmol/l) salicylic acid is in molar excess compared with albumin and only a small amount is bound. There is evidence that salicylic acid and aspirin share the same binding site on the lysine residue of the albumin. Studies of protein binding have led to the suggestion that both aspirin and salicylic acid may act by displacing a naturally occurring anti-inflammatory substance such as L-tryptophan or cortisol. However, there is little evidence to support this hypothesis. Indeed, no difference has been shown in the binding capacity of salicylic acid to serum albumin in patients with rheumatoid and osteo arthritis.

The ability of salicylic acid to bind to protein in the synovial fluid is considerably lower than it is in plasma, leading to lower concentrations of total drug. Aspirin concentrations are also significantly lower in synovial fliud, but peak much later and appear to be maintained for longer than those in plasma.

Salicylic acid concentrations in saliva reflect those of the plasma, but tend to vary with the pH at the site of production of saliva. Owing to this they should not be used for routine monitoring.

Salicylates diffuse slowly into CSF and it is likely that some of their analgesic and anti-pyretic effects are due to a direct influence on the hypothalamus. Likewise, both salicylic acid and aspirin readily cross the placental barrier, but although several studies in animals have shown an association between high doses and foetal abnormality, a number of prospective studies have failed to confirm teratogenicity in humans. Nevertheless, there is some evidence that chronic salicylate ingestion is associated with significantly reduced birthweight and an increase in perinatal mortality, haemorrhage and prolonged gestation. Foetal plasma concentrations are considerably higher than maternal plasma concentrations at birth. Salicylic acid is also found in breast milk and the potential exists for considerable exposure to salicylate in a child whose mother is maintained on doses administered for the treatment of rheumatoid arthritis.

Metabolism

A significant proportion (70%) of ingested aspirin reaches the systemic circulation. The remainder is hydrolysed to salicylic acid by non-specific esterases in the gut wall, plasma and liver. Plasma concentrations of aspirin rise rapidly after oral absorption, peak concentrations being achieved within 30 minutes of ingestion of soluble aspirin or 6 hours after the ingestion of enteric-coated preparations. Concentrations of aspirin in the plasma decline rapidly after peak values have been achieved. Aspirin elimination kinetics, after intravenous administration, are bi-exponential. The half-life of the first component is 2 to 5 minutes and that of the second 15 minutes. The hydrolysis of aspirin to salicylic acid is achieved rapidly *in vitro* (15 to 20 minutes) by the esterases present in human plasma. There appear to be clinically significant age- and sex-related differences in aspirin-esterase activity from various tissues and activity is reduced in patients with alcoholic liver disease. This may account for the variation in aspirin pharmacokinetics seen in individuals and certain disease states.

Once aspirin has been converted to salicylic acid it is removed from the body in one of five different ways. It can be excreted unchanged in the urine, conjugated with glycine to yield salicyluric acid, conjugated to form two glucuronides, salicylacyl glucuronide and salicyl phenolic glucuronide, respectively, and hydroxylated to form gentisic acid. Salicyluric acid and salicyl-phenolic

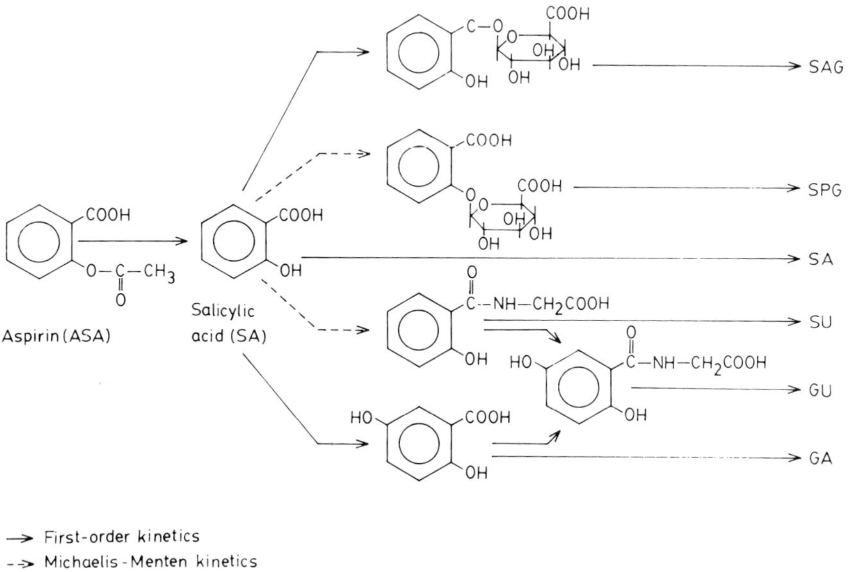

Figure 4.2. Metabolic pathways of acetylsalicylic and salicylic acids.

SAG — Salicyl-acyl glucuronide
SPG — Salicyl-phenolic glucuronide
SA — Salicylic acid
SU — Salicyluric acid
GU — Gentisuric acid
GA — Gentisic acid

glucuronide are formed by easily saturable Michaelis–Menten kinetics, while the other chemical reactions follow first-order kinetics. The pathways and their respective rate constants are shown in figure 4.2. Steady-state aspirin concentrations increase more than proportionately with an increase in dose, such that a daily increase from 2 to 4 g will lead to a fourfold increase in total plasma salicylate. As the daily dose increases, so more time is required to reach steady-state plasma concentration. Recently, it has been suggested that salicylic acid may induce its own metabolism by increasing the production of salicylurate. This would lead to the decline in steady-state plasma concentration which occurs during the first two weeks of salicylate use. The peak concentration of salicylacyl glucuronide is achieved at the same time as the peak concentration of free salicylic acid, but the salicyl-phenolic-glucuronide peak is delayed for eight hours. The formation of salicyl-phenolic glucuronide is capacity limited, but this has not been demonstrated for the other metabolites.

The half-life of elimination of salicylic acid varies from 3 hours at low dose (1 g) to 16 to 20 hours at recommended anti-inflammatory doses (3 to 6 g/day), and a number of trials have demonstrated that adequate steady-state concentrations of plasma salicylate can be maintained in patients with rheumatoid arthritis by administering salicylate twice daily. Since the protein binding of salicylic acid is dependent on concentration it tends to offset the non-linear elimination such that the total clearance remains largely unchanged. Consequently, the total concentration in plasma does not increase in quite the manner anticipated.

Free salicylic acid diffuses rapidly across the glomerulus and is actively secreted by the proximal tubule. The renal excretion of salicylic acid follows first-order kinetics and is extremely sensitive to urinary pH, the presence of urinary organic acids and urinary flow rate. The effect of change in urinary pH on salicylic acid clearance is most marked at high concentrations and may be important when patients are taking antacids likely to alter urinary pH. The renal excretion of salicylic acid is also reduced by probenecid which competes for secretion in the proximal tubule. The excretion of the conjugates is dependent on glomerular filtration and tubular secretion, but gentisic acid is excreted in the same way as free salicylic acid.

Clinical effects

Despite the widespread use of aspirin as an anti-pyretic and analgesic, it was not until 1965 that Fremont-Smith and Bayles demonstrated that doses between 3.6 and 7.5 g/day reduced proximal interphalangeal joint swelling and increased the range of movement and grip strength in patients with rheumatoid arthritis. Acetylsalicylic acid has both anti-inflammatory and analgesic effects in patients with arthritis, but the dose required to achieve an anti-inflammatory effect is in excess of 3 g/day.

A number of trials have compared aspirin with the newer NSAIDs. These studies indicate that aspirin is one of the most poorly tolerated NSAIDs, in terms of side-effects, and that it should no longer be the drug of first choice.

Although there is some evidence to suggest that aspirin may be a better anti-inflammatory and analgesic than salicylic acid, a recent study comparing choline magnesium trisalicylate and acetylsalicylic acid, in patients with rheumatoid arthritis, failed to demonstrate any significant difference in anti-inflammatory effect over a seven-week period. However, the incidence of side-effects was greater in the aspirin-treated group which also had the highest number of drop-outs.

Side-effects

Dyspepsia is still the most common side-effect reported by patients taking aspirin, and the exact relationship between aspirin ingestion and dyspepsia or peptic ulceration remains one of the great controversies of medicine. The advent of the gastroscope has not made the situation any clearer in that many patients with rheumatoid arthritis have asymptomatic gastric erosions and small ulcers, which may or may not be related to NSAID therapy. The standard method for measuring gastric blood loss is the chromium-51 red-cell-excretion technique. However, this cannot distinguish between blood loss from other areas in the gut and does not take into account biliary excrction. Indeed, chromium is excreted in the bile and aspirin increases biliary excretion thus confounding any possible interpretation of the results. There seems good evidence that enteric-coated or slow-release preparations reduce both symptomatic dyspepsia and chromium-51 blood loss, and should be the salicylates of first choice for the management of chronic rheumatic disease.

Although there is some epidemiological evidence to link aspirin intake with gastro-intestinal haemorrhage and peptic ulceration, the association is not strong and it is likely that a significant variation in response occurs between patients. According to recent evidence, there is a certain amount of gastric adaptation to aspirin and, from a practical point of view, peptic ulcers have been shown to heal in patients with rheumatoid arthritis despite continued salicylate therapy. The H2-blocking drugs (cimetidine and ranitidine) may aid the situation, but a past history of gastric ulceration, related to the salicylates, may not be as strong a contra-indication to further NSAID therapy as was once thought.

While the association between compound analgesic abuse and analgesic nephropathy is well known, there is conflicting evidence supporting the association between long-term salicylate ingestion and renal disease in patients with rheumatoid arthritis. Although acute changes in renal physiology, including reduced renal blood flow and increased white cell excretion, can be demonstrated, the patient's condition often reverts to normal despite continuing salicylate therapy. Several long-term studies in patients with rheumatoid arthritis have failed to show a significant relationship between salicylate ingestion and renal insufficiency. On the other hand, pathological examination of the kidneys in patients with rheumatoid arthritis demonstrates changes consistent with analgesic nephropathy in up to 20% of cases. Acute effects of salicylate on renal function, particularly in those patients with compromised renal physiology, are much more important than the potential for analgesic nephropathy. For this reason, patients with underlying renal disease, and particularly those with systemic lupus erythematosus, should be monitored carefully when salicylate therapy is commenced.

Many patients treated with salicylates show a mild increase in liver enzymes. This transaminitis is noted particularly in children with systemic disease and patients with active systemic lupus erythematosus. Most patients are asymptomatic, but some develop symptoms which make it necessary to stop their therapy. However, liver biopsies, in this situation, have usually shown mild non-specific changes only. Thus, in practice, salicylates should be continued until a significant increase in activity occurs. If symptoms of 'transaminitis' are observed, another NSAID should be used or the dose lowered sufficiently to prevent recurrence.

Aspirin ingestion prolongs the bleeding time in healthy individuals, but this is not clinically significant except in those patients with an underlying haemostatic defect such as von Willebrand's disease or haemophilia. Indeed, the anti-platelet effect of aspirin has been used to advantage in cardiovascular and cerebrovascular diseases. Aspirin, either alone or with sulfinpyrazone, would seem to reduce both the risk of stroke and the infarction rate in patients with coronary-artery disease. It also helps to prevent arterial thrombosis in patients with haemodialysis shunts and gives added protection against peripheral thrombo-embolism, when combined with oral anti-coagulants, in patients with prosthetic heart valves. However, conflicting results emerge from studies investigating the prophylaxis of deep-vein thrombosis. All these studies suffer from the problem that the optimal dose of aspirin has not yet been determined and that differences are seen between males and females in the benefit they derive. It is likely also that multiple mechanisms, in addition to platelet adhesion, are involved in the genesis of atherosclerosis.

Although aspirin hypersensitivity is one of the most common allergic drug reactions it is extremely rare when one considers the amounts consumed worldwide. Allergy to aspirin can manifest in a number of ways — urticaria and angio-oedema, anaphylaxis or bronchospasm. Bronchospasm and urticaria with angio-oedema are the most common reactions seen and those developing bronchospasm often have associated nasal polyps. Increased IgE concentrations and eosinophilia are sometimes seen, suggesting a true allergic phenomenon, as is an imbalance of bronchoconstrictor and bronchodilator prostaglandins, which can be corrected by administering disodium cromoglycate.

Hypersensitivity is relatively rare in rheumatological practice, but aspirin-induced attacks occur in about 10% of patients who have asthma. If asthmatic attacks are induced, care should be taken in the prescription of other NSAIDs. Interestingly, the fenamates can often be used when all else fails as they do not induce asthmatic attacks owing to their antagonism of the bronchoconstrictor prostaglandin PGF.

Aspirin and salicylates, like other prostaglandin inhibitors, can provoke sodium retention and cause the development of pulmonary and peripheral oedema. Thus, care should be taken when prescribing large doses of salicylate to elderly patients with underlying coronary-artery disease.

Drug interactions

The potential for drug interactions is vast because the salicylates are widely prescribed. Antacids are commonly prescribed with aspirin, but will influence salicylic acid concentrations only when large doses (in excess of 100 ml/day)

Table 4.2. Interactions of salicylates.

Interacting drug	**Effect**
Antacids (absorbable > 100 ml/day)	Increase excretion of salicylic acid
Indomethacin	Variable reported effects on plasma concentrations
Propionic-acid derivatives	
Fenoprofen	Reduced plasma concentrations of fenoprofen
Naproxen	Reduced plasma concentrations of naproxen
Flubiprofen	Reduced plasma concentrations of flurbiprofen
Ibuprofen	Reduced plasma concentrations of ibuprofen
Ketoprofen	Reduced plasma concentrations of ketoprofen
Diflunisal	Reduced diflunisal concentrations
Diclofenac	Reduced diclofenac concentrations
Phenylbutazone	Reduced uricosuria induced by high-dose salicylic acid
Sulphinpyrazone	
Sulphonylurea hypoglycaemic agents	Effect potentiated by high-dose salicylic acid
Corticosteroids	Variable effect (possible induction of salicylic acid metabolism by corticosteroids).

are taken. Salicylates are still commonly prescribed with other NSAIDs and give rise to a number of pharmacokinetic interactions (table 4.2). They have little effect on the plasma concentrations of indomethacin, but will reduce the plasma concentrations of a number of other NSAIDs. The clinical effect of this reduction is unclear, but does not appear to be of any real significance. However, it is possible that side-effects are more common when two NSAIDs are taken together. The uricosuria induced by high doses of salicylic acid is reduced by phenylbutazone, probenecid and sulfinpyrazone. High doses of salicylates may potentiate the hypoglycaemic effects of oral anti-diabetic agents. There has been some suggestion that the metabolism of the salicylates can be induced by corticosteroids, since plasma concentrations of salicylate have been shown to increase in patients when the dose of corticosteroid is reduced. However, controlled studies to assess this interaction have failed to show any significant effect. The renal clearance of methotrexate is significantly inhibited by salicylate and it may also be displaced from its binding sites. Thus, care should be taken when these two drugs are administered concurrently. Phenytoin is also displaced from its binding sites by salicylate, but the free concentrations are not significantly altered and no dosage adjustment needs to be made. Interactions may well occur between salicylates and diuretic and hypotensive agents, as these drugs may act in part through prostaglandin-mediated mechanisms. The mechanisms of many drug interactions seen with salicylates are complex and are often not pharmacokinetically mediated. Therefore, care should be taken whenever salicylates are prescribed with other drugs.

Further reading

Atkinson, D. C. and Collier, H. T., 1980, Salicylates: molecular mechanisms of therapeutic action. *Advances in Pharmacology and Chemotherapy*, **17**, 233–288.

Barnett, H. J. M., Hirsch, J. and Mustard, J. F., 1982, *Acetylsalicylic Acid: New Uses for an Old Drug*. Raven Press, New York.

Buchanan, W. W., Rooney, P. J. and Rennie, J. A. N., 1979, Aspirin and the salicylates. *Clinics in Rheumatic Diseases*, **5**, 499–539.

Day, R. O., Graham, G. G., Champion, G. D. and Lee, E., 1983, Clinically significant drug interactions with anti-rheumatic drugs. In *Anti-rheumatic Drugs. Clinical Pharmacology and Therapeutics*, Volume 3. Edited E. C. Huskisson, (Praeger) pp. 37–54.

Levy, G., 1979, Pharmacokinetics of salicylates in man. *Drug Metabolism Reviews*, **9**, 3–19.

Needs, C. J. and Brooks, P. M., 1985, Clinical pharmacokinetics of the salicylates. *Clinical Pharmacokinetics*, **10**, 164–177.

5. Non-steroidal anti-inflammatory drugs

The NSAIDs form the basis of treatment for inflammatory polyarthritis. Since the isolation of the active component of willow bark and subsequent development of chemical methods for producing salicylic acid and aspirin, the importance of having relatively safe drugs to suppress pain and inflammation has been appreciated. In the latter part of the last century pyrazole derivatives were used as analgesic, anti-pyretic and anti-inflammatory agents and this led to the developments of phenylbutazone and oxyphenbutazone. In the 1960s, indomethacin was introduced and was followed by a new group of NSAIDs, the propionic-acid derivatives. Many different chemical classes of NSAIDs are now available (table 5.1) and their pharmacology, pharmacokinetics and clinical use will be discussed in this chapter. These drugs make up one of the largest groups of pharmacological agents prescribed worldwide and it has been estimated that, in 1984, the cost of drugs of this class, excluding salicylates, was in excess of two billion US dollars. With the increasing age of the population it is likely that the market for this group of drugs will continue to increase, providing a stimulus for the pharmaceutical industry to develop new agents in this class.

The carboxy- and heterocyclic-acetic acids

Indomethacin

The chemical structure of indomethacin (1-(*p*-chlorobenzoyl)-5-methoxy-2-methylindole-3-acetic acid) is shown in figure 5.1. Although indomethacin is virtually insoluble in water, it is stable in a number of alcohols and aqueous buffers at pH 7.5. The analgesic, anti-pyretic and anti-inflammatory effects of indomethacin can be demonstrated in a variety of animal models, including the cotton-pellet granuloma model, adjuvant arthritis, carrageenan-induced oedema and the rabbit ear model. The major mechanism of action appears to be reversible inhibition of the enzyme cyclo-oxygenase. Cyclo-oxygenase has a binding site which can be occupied by a lipid component of indomethacin, thus preventing the enzyme from working. Indomethacin has been shown to inhibit both the chemotactic and chemokinetic responses of neutrophils and to

Table 5.1. Classification of non-steroidal anti-inflammatory drugs.

Carboxylic acids	Salicylic acids and esters		Aspirin, Diflunisal, Benorylate
	Acetic acids	Phenylacetic	Diclofenac, Alcofenac, Fenclofenac
		Carbo- and heterocyclic acetic acids	Indomethacin, Sulindac, Tolmetin
	Propionic acids		Ibuprofen, Flurbiprofen, Naproxen, Ketoprofen, Fenoprofen, Fenbufen, Indoprofen, Suprofen, Tiaprofen, Pirprofen
	Fenamic acids		Mefenamic, Flufenamic, Meclofenamic, Niflumic
Enolic acids	Pyrazolones		Oxyphenbutazone, Phenylbutazone, Feprazone, Azapropazone
	Oxicams		Piroxicam, Sudoxicam, Isoxicam

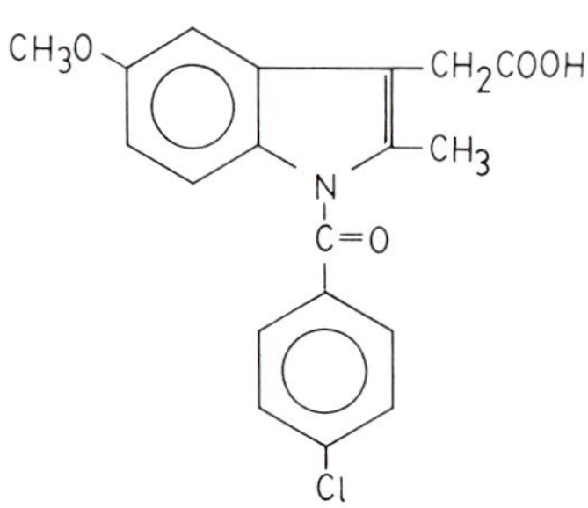

Figure 5.1. The structure of indomethacin.

stabilize lysosomal membranes. Whether this is due to a direct effect of indomethacin or to the suppression of arachidonic-acid metabolism is not clear.

Indomethacin is rapidly and completely absorbed following oral administration, with peak plasma concentrations being achieved 1 to 1.5 hours after administration. Taking indomethacin with meals delays its absorption, but does not affect bioavailability. Recently, sustained-release preparations of indomethacin have been produced which produce lower peak plasma concentrations and less variable and more sustained concentrations than standard preparation. To reduce gastric irritation, indomethacin can be administered rectally, and although peak plasma concentrations are usually attained sooner, they are usually lower than those seen following oral administration.

Indomethacin is largely bound to plasma proteins (90–98%) and is widely distributed to body tissues. The apparent volume of distribution of indomethacin is between 0.15 and 0.2 l/kg. Indomethacin enters synovial fluid slowly, crosses the placental barrier and is found in low concentrations in breast milk. It is metabolized by a variety of means, including demethylation, deacylation and glucuronidation. The parent compound and its major metabolites are largely excreted in the urine and faeces. Indomethacin undergoes extensive entero-hepatic re-circulation. About 10% is conjugated with glucuronic acid by hepatic microsomal enzymes and is excreted into the bile, where it is resorped after hydrolysis. This recycling process is thought to account for the marked variability in pharmacokinetic studies, where the plasma elimination half-life of indomethacin has been reported anywhere between 1 and 16 hours.

Indomethacin has been shown to be efficacious in the treatment of rheumatoid arthritis, ankylosing spondylitis, osteoarthritis, gout, juvenile rheumatoid arthritis, acute soft-tissue rheumatism and dysmenorrhoea. Like other NSAIDs, it has also been useful as an anti-pyretic and analgesic in treating symptoms associated with neoplastic disease (fever, bone pain, and hypercalcaemia), and a variety of other conditions including pericarditis, uveitis, and Bartter's syndrome. Indomethacin at high doses (300–400 mg in the first 24 hours) is particularly useful in the initial stages of the treatment of acute gout. The dose of indomethacin is then reduced to 100–150 mg daily and maintained for 1–2 weeks. Interestingly patients with gout on these high dose regimens do not seem to suffer from side effects. Indomethacin is used as the drug of choice for the treatment of ankylosing spondylitis and other sero-negative spondyloarthropathies. Many comparative trials have shown it to be an effective agent for suppressing pain and inflammation in chronic rheumatoid arthritis. When given, either as a suppository or a large oral dose at night, it is particularly useful in alleviating morning stiffness and night pain. In the treatment of osteoarthritis, controlled studies against newer NSAIDs show no difference between the drugs in terms of pain relief, but the newer drugs tend to produce less side-effects.

About 30% of patients taking indomethacin will suffer an adverse reaction.

Although most of these are mild, in 15–20% of patients they are likely to lead to cessation of therapy. The major side-effects are gastro-intestinal, with nausea and dyspepsia being most common. Central nervous system side-effects, including headache and dizziness, are frequently reported also. Sodium retention leading to oedema, increased blood pressure and weight gain, and the occasional occurrrence of haematological problems (leucopaenia, bone-marrow depression and thrombocytopaenia) are unusual, but the prescribing physician needs to be aware of their possible occurrence.

Since indomethacin is commonly prescribed its potential for interaction with concomitantly prescribed drugs is high. Some antacid preparations, such as magnesium and aluminium hydroxide, delay the absorption of indomethacin, but do not effect the total bioavailability. Indomethacin does not have any affect on prothrombin time in patients treated with warfarin, but combinations of NSAIDs and anti-coagulants should be viewed with caution because of the effect of NSAIDs on platelet function and their potential for gastric erosion. The hypotensive effects of a number of drugs including propranolol, hydralazine, captopril and other beta-adrenergic blocking drugs are reduced by indomethacin. In addition, both the natriuretic and diuretic effects of frusemide and the thiazides are attenuated and this may have important clinical implications in the elderly patient. Probenecid inhibits the metabolic clearance of indomethacin by interfering with glucuronidation and this leads to increased plasma concentrations of indomethacin and an enhanced anti-inflammatory effect, but no increase in toxicity.

Indomethacin is particularly useful in the treatment of active inflammation, both acute and chronic, and is available in the following forms—25 and 50 mg capsules, 50 and 100 mg suppositories, 75 mg sustained-release capsule, 5 mg/ml oral suspension and an intramuscular preparation 50 mg/2 ml solution. Most patients achieve a clinical response with a total daily dose of 150 mg or less.

Sulindac

Sulindac is (Z)-5-fluoro-2-methyl-1,1-[*p*-(methyl-sulphinyl) phenyl]methylene-1H-indene-3-acetic acid. It is moderately soluble in water at neutral and alkaline pH and is converted to a biologically inactive sulphone, and the biologically active sulphide *in vivo*. The formulae and reaction are shown in figure 5.2.

Both sulindac and its sulphide have been shown to have analgesic, anti-inflammatory and anti-pyretic properties in a variety of animal models. In these systems the sulphide is much more potent than the parent compound. In contrast to indomethacin, the sulphide interferes both with the cyclo-oxygenase and lipoxygenase pathways of arachidonic-acid metabolism and can act as a scavenger of oxygen radicals. Sulindac is rapidly absorbed following oral administration, with peak plasma concentrations of both sulindac and its

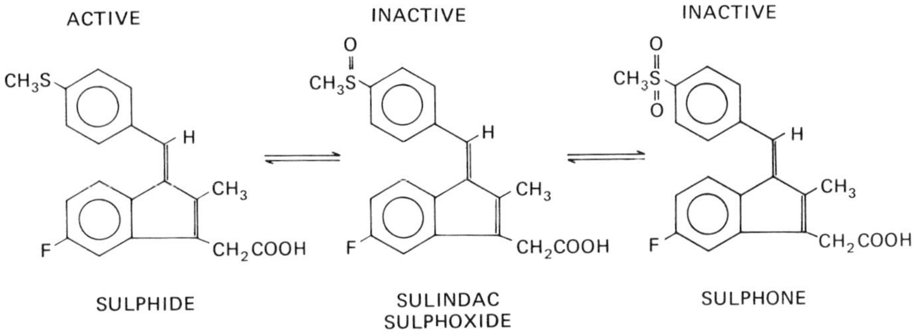

Figure 5.2. Sulindac and its metabolites.

active sulphide being seen within two hours of administration. Although oral bioavailability is high, both the rate and extent of absorption are reduced when the drug is taken with food. The plasma protein binding of sulindac and its sulphide metabolite are in excess of 90%. Sulindac is reversibly oxidized to the inactive sulphone or reduced to sulindac sulphide, the active metabolite. The sulphone is eliminated after glucuronidation, by urinary and faecal excretion. Sulindac, its sulphone and active sulphide all undergo intra-hepatic circulation in man, although the active sulphide is not metabolized to the same extent as the parent compound and the sulphone. The sulphide metabolite is eliminated directly in the faeces, following biliary excretion, or re-oxidized to sulindac. The complex disposition of sulindac prevents any conventional analysis of its pharmacokinetics being made from accumulation studies. However, mean effective elimination half-lives of eight hours for sulindac and 16 hours for the sulphide can be deduced. Total-body content of the active sulphide tends to be conserved through the process of reversible metabolism, the enterohepatic circulation of sulindac and the relative absence of renal excretion of the sulphide. The exposure of the gastric mucosa to the active sulphide is minimal because sulindac and its sulphone are the principal species undergoing intrahepatic circulation and the sulphide is not excreted in the urine. These pharmacokinetic properties may well explain the relatively low incidence of gastric and renal side-effects seen with sulindac. It has been shown that, in contrast to indomethacin, sulindac does not modify urinary prostaglandin excretion and plasma renin activity or block frusemide-induced renin release. This effect may be produced if renal cyclo-oxygenase is less sensitive to inhibition by the sulphide or if the sulphide is differenterially distributed and formed within the kidney. These properties may explain the relative lack of effect of sulindac in patients with renal impairment.

Clinical efficacy of sulindac has been shown in osteoarthritis, soft-tissue rheumatism, acute gout, ankylosing spondylitis and rheumatoid arthritis. The drug is well tolerated in doses of 200 to 400 mg/day and has similar effects to other NSAIDs. Adverse reactions occur in less than 10% of patients and include abdominal pain, nausea, constipation and occasional headache and dizziness. Liver-enzyme concentrations are sometimes elevated and occasionally patients are jaundiced and have evidence of cholestasis or hepatitis. No interactions have been reported between sulindac and antacids, warfarin or sulphonylurea-hypoglycaemic agents.

Sulindac is an effective anti-inflammatory analgesic agent and may be particularly valuable in patients with mild renal insufficiency. Sulindac is available in 100 mg and 200 mg tablets and as 200 mg suppositories. The usual dose is 200–400 mg/day given once or twice daily.

Tolmetin

The acetic acid derivative, tolmetin sodium, [*N*-methyl-5-(*p*-toluoyl)-pyrrole-2-acetate dihydrate], is structurally related to indomethacin, with a pyrrole ring substituted for the indole nucleus (figure 5.3). This compound has been shown to have analgesic, anti-pyretic and anti-inflammatory activity in a variety of animal models, including carrageenan- and kaolin-induced rat-paw oedema, adjuvant arthritis and ultraviolet-induced erythema. It reversibly inhibits cyclo-oxygenase leading to the suppression of prostaglandin production.

Tolmetin sodium is rapidly and almost completely absorbed following oral administration with peak plasma concentrations being achieved within 60 minutes. It is largely bound to plasma proteins and eliminated primarily by renal excretion of its oxidative metabolite. About 17% of an oral dose is excreted unchanged, the rest being recovered as glucuronide or other minor metabolites. Tolmetin has a short plasma half-life of between five and six hours and does not show any accumulation on chronic administration.

As a drug it is efficacious in rheumatoid arthritis, juvenile arthritis, osteo-arthritis, ankylosing spondylitis and soft-tissue rheumatism. Comparative studies have shown it to be well tolerated and of similar efficacy to other NSAIDs.

The administration of magnesium aluminium hydroxide gel with tolmetin has no significant effect on peak plasma concentrations or bioavailability, but concomitant aspirin administration reduces plasma concentration, possibly displacing tolmetin from its protein binding sites. No significant interaction has been demonstrated between tolmetin sodium and warfarin, or phenpro-coumon, insulin or oral hypoglycaemic agents.

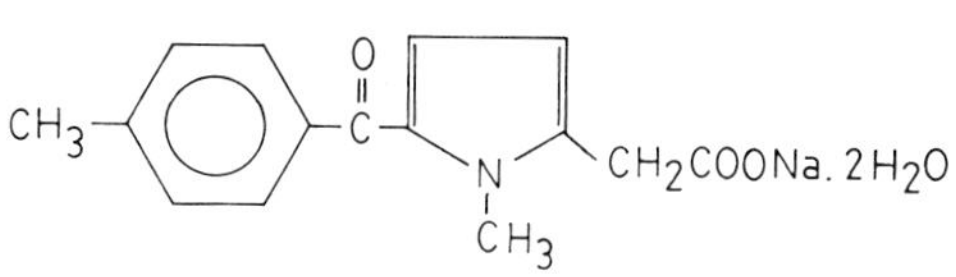

Figure 5.3. Tolmetin sodium.

Tolmetin sodium is well tolerated during both short- and long-term therapy with the most frequent side-effects being gastro-intestinal or neurological. Symptoms in most patients are controlled with doses of between 600 and 1800 mg/day administered in three equally divided doses. In juvenile rheumatoid arthritis, therapy can be initiated with a dose of 20 mg/day, increasing to 30 mg/kg/day given as three or four divided doses.

Phenylacetic acid derivatives

Diclofenac

Diclofenac, sodium {*O*-[(2,6-dichlorophenyl)-amino]-phenyl}-acetate, has been shown to have anti-pyretic, analgesic and anti-inflammatory effects on a variety of animal models including yeast-induced fever, carrageenan- and kaolin-induced oedema and adjuvant arthritis. It is a potent inhibitor of prostaglandin-synthetase activity, inhibits the release of lysosomal enzymes (cathepsin B and neutral protease) and platelet aggregation. Its structure is shown in figure 5.4.

Diclofenac sodium is rapidly absorbed after oral administration with maximum concentrations being achieved between 0.5 and 1.5 hours after administration of an enteric-coated tablet. Food delays the absorption of a single dose, but has little effect on the total amount absorbed. Diclofenac is also absorbed rectally at a rate similar to that of oral administration.

Diclofenac is strongly bound to plasma proteins (greater than 99%) and has a low apparent volume of distribution (0.12 l/kg) It is extensively metabolized by hydroxylation, conjugated with glucuronic acid and taurineamide, or excreted as conjugates of the hydroxylated derivatives. In man, although biliary excretion occurs, most is excreted renally. The elimination is bi-phasic with a terminal elimination half-life of about one hour. Pharmacokinetic studies indicate that there is no saturation of distribution or metabolism over

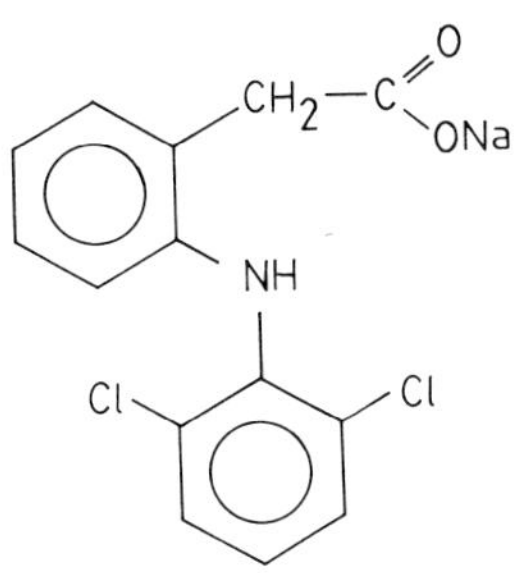

Figure 5.4. Diclofenac.

a dose range of 25–150 mg and there is no evidence to suggest a change in metabolism with time. Diclofenac sodium enters the synovial fluid compartment slowly and concentrations remain relatively constant on chronic dosing, although steady-state plasma concentrations cannot be achieved owing to its short half-life.

In the treatment of rheumatoid arthritis, diclofenac sodium has been shown to be better than a placebo and of comparable efficacy to indomethacin, aspirin, ibuprofen, phenylbutazone and naproxen. It is no different to indomethacin, aspirin, ibuprofen, and naproxen in the treatment of osteoarthritis, although well tolerated, and is useful in the treatment of ankylosing spondylitis, acute gout and psoriatic arthropathy. Long-term studies in both rheumatoid and osteoarthritis indicate low incidence of side-effects, although those that do occur resemble the effects of other NSAIDs. Unusual side-effects include abnormalities of liver function, leucopaenia, thrombocytopaenia and aplastic anaemia.

Diclofenac sodium does seem to increase the effect of oral anti-coagulants, but the risk of haemorrhage is low. It does not alter thyroid function in euthyroid rheumatoid patients. Aspirin reduces plasma drug concentrations probably by increasing biliary excretion and altering drug distribution. It is not known whether this decrease has any clinical significance. Diclofenac sodium does not alter the effect of oral hypoglycaemic agents. Studies in elderly patients and those with renal failure have failed to demonstrate any significant change in pharmacokinetics with age, but have shown the excretion of diclofenac and its metabolites in the urine to be related to glomerular-filtration rate. In renal insufficiency the plasma concentration of diclofenac is not altered although the concentrations of the inactive metabolites tend to be elevated.

Diclofenac sodium is available in 25 and 50 mg enteric-coated tablets, as a 50 mg suppository and as an intramuscular injection (50 mg/ml). The dose of diclofenac is between 50 and 150 mg/day administered two or three times daily.

Fenclofenac

Fenclofenac, 2-(2,4-dichlorophenoxy)phenylacetic acid, (figure 5.5) was first synthesized in 1967 and has been shown to have analgesic, anti-pyretic and anti-inflammatory activity in standard model systems. It is a comparatively weak inhibitor of cyclo-oxygenase and seems to act rather differently from other NSAIDs against the cellular phase of delayed hypersensitivity.

Fenclofenac is rapidly absorbed after oral administration, with peak plasma concentrations being achieved in three to four hours. It is strongly bound to plasma proteins (greater than 99%), particularly albumin, but also binds to thyroid-binding globulin and consequently interferes with competitive-binding assays for thyroid hormones. Although thyroid function is unaffected by

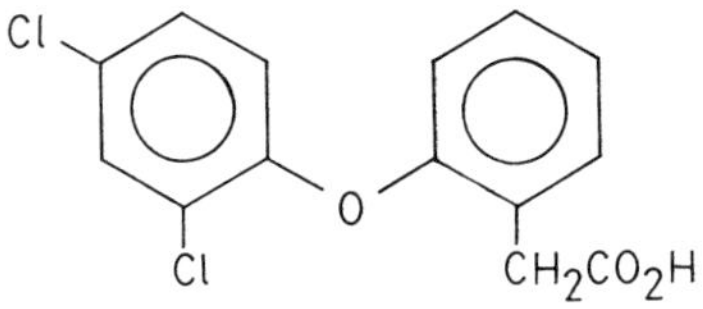

Figure 5.5. Fenclofenac.

fenclofenac therapy, the competition for protein binding reduces the plasma concentrations of T3 and T4. The major metabolic pathway for fenclofenac in man is glucuronidation and although some biliary excretion occurs, intrahepatic circulation is of minor importance in man. Drug metabolism occurs in the liver with subsequent renal excretion. Pharmacokinetic studies reveal a terminal half-life of between 20 and 38 hours with no evidence of dose-dependent kinetics in daily doses of up to 1800 mg.

Fenclofenac has been shown to be efficacious in the treatment of rheumatoid arthritis, osteoarthritis, ankylosing spondylitis and soft-tissue injuries. It has also been used in a small number of children with juvenile chronic arthritis where it has controlled disease activity and shown acceptable tolerance. In a large study 25% of patients reported gastro-intestinal and 18.9% dermatological side-effects. Skin rashes, however, resulted in the highest percentage of patients withdrawing from the study (10.2%). Observations of an anti-rheumatic effect in animals led to clinical trials which indicated that fenclofenac had similar activity to D-penicillamine and gold in patients with rheumatoid disease. Further studies comparing fenclofenac with other SAARDs and examining its influence on joint erosion are currently being investigated.

The recommended dose of fenclofenac is 900–1800 mg/day given in divided doses.

Propionic acid derivatives

The arylpropionic acid derivatives ibuprofen, flurbiprofen, naproxen, fenoprofen, ketoprofen, indoprofen and suprofen and the thienyl analogue tiaprofenic acid are chiral: they exist in two structurally different forms known as enantiomers which are mirror images of each other. These drugs are administered as racemates (mixtures of enantiomers) except in the case of naproxen. The symbolism refers to *R* (rectus) or *S* (sinister) which nominates the chiral form. The major anti-inflammatory and analgesic activity is contained in the *S* form but the *R* form maybe weakly active. One way transformation of *R* to *S* occurs *in vivo* in man and differential rates of transformation may explain some of the variability in response noted clinically. For example, if there is drug accumulation as might occur in renal insufficiency, more *R* to *S* inversion may occur than would with normal renal function.

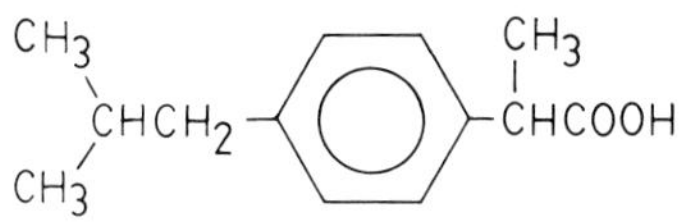

Figure 5.6. Ibuprofen.

Ibuprofen

Ibuprofen, *RS*-2-(4-isobutylphenyl)propionic acid (figure 5.6), was introduced into clinical practice in 1969. In standard animal models it has anti-pyretic, analgesic and anti-inflammatory effects. It inhibits cyclo-oxygenase, stabilizes proteins against denaturation by heat, antagonizes leucocyte adherence and chemotaxis and inhibits superoxide-ion production.

Ibuprofen is rapidly absorbed and peak plasma concentrations are seen within two hours of oral administration. This peak may be reduced by food, but the total bioavailability is not significantly altered. Ibuprofen is largely bound to plasma proteins (greater than 99%) and passes slowly into the synovial fluid where, three hours after oral administration, it attains concentrations higher than those of plasma. Ibuprofen is eliminated primarily by biotransformation and urinary excretion with an elimination half-life of approximately 2.5 hours.

Ibuprofen is efficacious in the treatment of rheumatoid arthritis, osteoarthritis, juvenile chronic polyarthritis, and non-articular rheumatism or soft-tissue injury. As a result of clinical experience, the recommended daily dose has risen from 800 mg to 2.4 g and some patients tolerate 3.6 g without significant ill effect. A controlled clinical trial found little difference between doses of 1.6 and 2.4 g/day although dose-related responses were apparent at lower doses. Owing to its low incidence of side-effects, ibuprofen has been approved for over-the-counter prescribing in the United States and Great Britain. The side-effects are those of other NSAIDs (gastrointestinal and allergic rashes). A few individuals have been reported to have developed toxic amblyopia with ibuprofen therapy, but several large series have failed to confirm any association. Plasma ibuprofen concentrations are reduced by concurrent salicylate therapy, but ibuprofen has no effect on oral anti-coagulant therapy. Ibuprofen decreases creatinine clearance and increases serum creatinine in some patients with chronic glomerulonephiritis, thus, care must be taken when prescribing ibuprofen to patients with compromised renal function.

Ibuprofen is available in 200 and 400 mg tablets and as a suspension. The recommended dose is 1.2–1.6 g/day in many countries, but a dose of 2.4 g/day is approved in the United States.

Flurbiprofen

The structure of flurbiprofen, *RS*-[2-(2-fluoro-4-biphenylyl)]propionic acid, is shown in figure 5.7. This drug has potent anti-pyretic analgesic and anti-

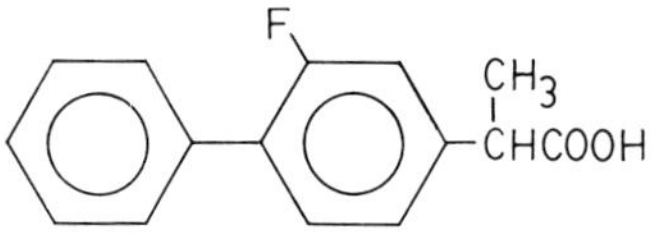

Figure 5.7. Flurbiprofen.

inflammatory effects in animal models, inhibits platelet aggregation and suppresses prostaglandin synthesis and leucocyte migration.

Peak plasma concentrations are achieved within 1.5 hours of an oral dose and are reduced by food. Suppositories show similar bioavailability to tablets. The drug is strongly bound to plasma proteins and is readily distributed to synovial fluid. It undergoes biotransformation and both parent compound and metabolites are excreted renally. The rate of elimination of flurbiprofen is slightly slower than that of ibuprofen, with a half-life of four hours. Repeated dosing of flurbiprofen has no effect on pharmacokinetic parameters and although strongly bound to plasma proteins, less than 10% of the binding capacity is occupied making protein-binding interactions unlikely. Flurbiprofen is effective in the treatment of rheumatoid arthritis, osteroarthritis, ankylosing spondylitis and as an analgesic in patients with post-operative pain or sports injuries. It is well tolerated by all age groups and the pattern of side-effects is similar to that of other NSAIDs. The plasma concentration of flurbiprofen is reduced by concurrent salicylate therapy. There is no significant interaction with oral anti-coagulants, but the diuretic effect of frusemide is attenuated. The dose of flurbiprofen is between 150 and 300 mg/day and can be given as infrequently as twice daily.

Naproxen

Naproxen, *S*-2-(6-methoxy-2-naphthyl)propionic acid, (figure 5.8) has been shown to have analgesic, anti-pyretic and anti-inflammatory effects in a variety of animal models. It stabilizes lysosomal membranes *in vitro*, reduces neutrophil migration *in vitro* and *in vivo*, and is a potent inhibitor of cyclo-oxygenase.

Naproxen is rapidly absorbed after oral or rectal administration and peak plasma concentrations are achieved within two hours. Oral absorption is

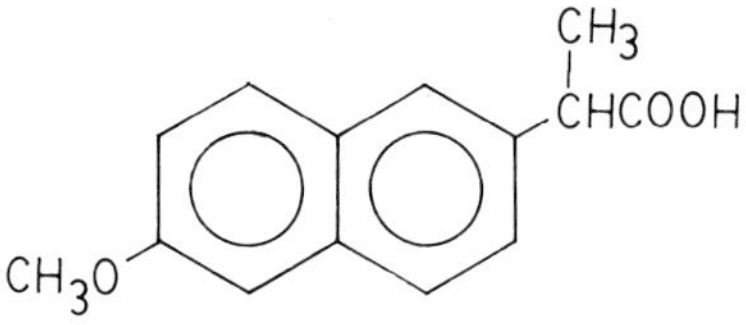

Figure 5.8. Naproxen.

somewhat delayed by food, although the total amount absorbed is unchanged. The sodium salt of naproxen is absorbed more rapidly than the free acid and may be particularly useful for analgesia. The binding of naproxen to plasma proteins is concentration dependent, ranging from 99.6%, at concentrations between 23 and 40 μg/ml to 97.4%, at concentrations of 473 μg/ml. Naproxen has a small volume of distribution (0.1 l/kg), crosses the placental barrier and is found at about 1% of the plasma concentration in the milk of lactating women. It is distributed slowly to the synovial fluid. Since protein binding is dependent on concentration, clearance of the drug is accelerated as the dose increases. The major pathway of elimination is by glucuronide conjugation; less than 10% of the ingested naproxen dose is excreted unchanged in the urine and faecal excretion is negligible. Naproxen has a long elimination half-life (about 13 hours) which is not altered by dose or duration of administration. Naproxen does not accumulate and its pharmacokinetics are not altered in patients with renal failure. Over the last decade this drug has been tested extensively in comparative controlled trials and has been found to be useful in the treatment of rheumatoid arthritis, osteoarthritis, ankylosing spondylitis, gout and juvenile rheumatoid arthritis. More recently its usefulness as an analgesic agent in the treatment of post-operative pain, soft-tissue rheumatism and dysmenorrhoea has been appreciated. It seems at least as effective as other NSAIDs in the treatment of pain and inflammation, and is often the preferred preparation in terms of pain relief and lack of side-effects. Recent studies have shown that many patients, particularly those with osteoarthritis, may be maintained on a single daily dose. In patients with rheumatoid arthritis, a relationship between serum naproxen concentration and efficacy has been observed over the range 250 to 1500 mg/day. Side-effects are similar to those of other NSAIDs, with gastro-intestinal symptoms being reported most commonly. Renal abnormalities, including interstitial nephritis, occasionally occur, but do not constitute a major problem. Rare side-effects such as thrombocytopaenia, skin rashes and jaundice have been reported.

Drug absorption is enhanced by sodium bicarbonate and reduced by magnesium oxide and aluminium hydroxide. The clinical importance of these interactions is unknown. Concurrent administration of aspirin produces a significant decrease in the concentration of plasma naproxen, but this effect does not appear to be clinically significant. Although naproxen increases the serum-free fraction of warfarin, this does not seem to be accompanied by a change in anti-coagulant activity. No significant interaction occurs between naproxen and tolbutamide. Probenecid significantly increases naproxen concentrations by interfering with glucuronidation. Concurrent cimetidine administration does not alter naproxen kinetics, or the H2-blocking action of cimetidine.

Naproxen is available in 250 and 500 mg tablets and as a suppository. The usual adult dose is in the region of 500 to 750 mg/day, but some patients may require up to 1.5 g to achieve adequate pain relief. The dosage should be

adjusted according to individual requirements and response, and can be administered once or twice daily.

Fenoprofen

Fenoprofen, *RS*-2-(3-phenoxyphenyl)propionic acid (figure 5.9), is produced as a calcium dihydrate salt and is a racemic mixture, there being no apparent difference between the pharmacological activities of the *R* and *S* isomers and the racemate. Anti-inflammatory, anti-pyretic and analgesic activities have been established in animal model systems.

Fenoprofen inhibits the release of prostaglandin from human platelets and synovial tissues by interfering with cyclo-oxygenase, reduces the release of acid hydrolases from leucocyte lysosomes and inhibits complement-mediated cell lysis and mitogen-stimulated lymphocyte responses.

Fenoprofen calcium is rapidly absorbed following oral administration, with peak plasma concentrations being achieved within two hours. The absorption of fenoprofen is reduced by food, but not antacids. Plasma concentrations increase linearly with doses up to 3.2 g/day and there is no change in kinetics with continuous dosing. The drug is strongly bound to plasma proteins and readily distributed to synovial fluid. The plasma elimination half-life is about three hours and the glucuronide metabolites are excreted by the kidney.

Fenoprofen calcium is useful (in doses of 2–4 g/day) in the treatment of rheumatoid arthritis, osteoarthritis, ankylosing spondylitis, acute gout and soft-tissue rheumatism. Adverse reactions are similar to those of the other NSAIDs, with gastro-intestinal side-effects being most common. Patients occasionally complain of headaches and other neurological side-effects, and interstitial nephritis and haematological conditions have also been reported.

The concurrent administration of salicylates reduces plasma concentrations as does phenobarbitone. Whether this has a clinical effect is not known.

Fenoprofen is available in 300 mg tablets and the standard recommended dose is 1.2–2.4 g/day. Some patients may require more than this to control their symptoms and the drug is usually given four times daily.

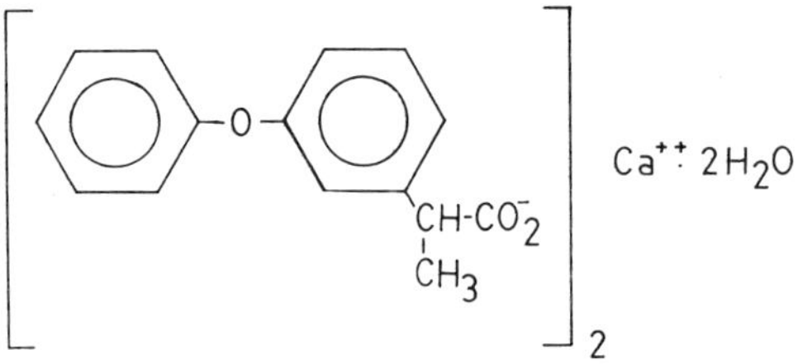

Figure 5.9. Fenoprofen.

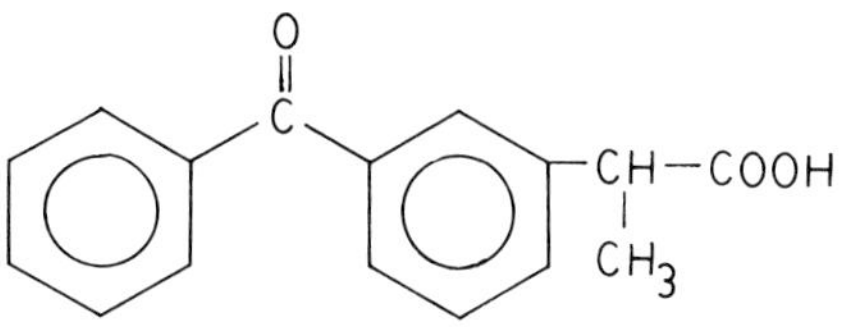

Figure 5.10. Ketoprofen.

Ketoprofen

Ketoprofen, *RS*-2-(3-benzoylphenyl)propionic acid (figure 5.10), was synthesized in 1967. Like most other propionic acids, it is practically insoluble in water. Ketoprofen has been shown to have analgesic, anti-pyretic and anti-inflammatory effects in animal models and, like other NSAIDs, inhibits prostaglandin production. It has also been shown to stabilize lysosomal membranes and to inhibit platelet aggregation both *in vitro* and *in vivo*.

Ketoprofen is rapidly absorbed following oral administration and peak plasma levels are achieved within 90 minutes. Stable plasma concentrations occur within 48 hours and there is no evidence of accumulation or alteration in pharmacokinetics with prolonged administration. The drug is strongly bound to plasma proteins, but readily enters the synovial fluid. The plasma half-life is in the region of 1.5 to 2 hours. Ketoprofen is metabolized primarily to glucuronic-acid derivatives and is then eliminated in the urine.

Ketoprofen is used in the treatment of rheumatoid arthritis, ankylosing spondylitis, osteoarthritis of the hip and knee, and acute gouty arthritis. A large number of open studies have suggested that it is effective in soft-tissue rheumatism too. Ketoprofen tends to be well tolerated in comparison to other NSAIDs, although similar side-effects occur, indigestion and nausea being the most common.

Probenecid increases plasma concentrations of ketoprofen, not only by reducing the renal clearance of unchanged ketoprofen, but also by affecting conjugation to the glucuronides. Whether this interaction has a clinical effect is unclear.

Ketoprofen is available in 25, 50 or 100 mg capsules, as a suppository (100 mg) or as a lyophilized preparation for intramuscular use. The usual dose is between 100 and 300 mg and this may be prescribed three or four times daily.

Indoprofen

Indoprofen, *RS*-α[4-(1-oxo-2-isoindolinyl)phenyl]propionic acid (figure 5.11), is a weak acid with a relatively low pK_a which circulates in the blood in an ionized form which precludes penetration of the blood–brain barrier. It has been shown to have anti-inflammatory, analgesic and anti-pyretic effects

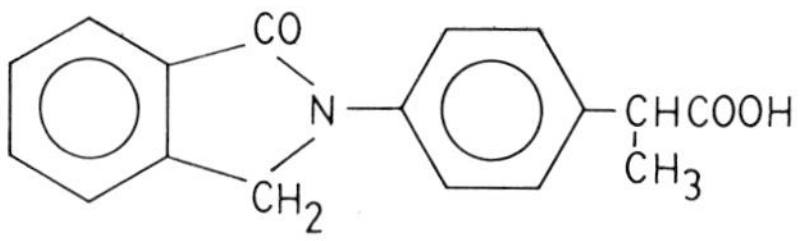

Figure 5.11. Indoprofen.

in animal models. Like other NSAIDs, it interferes with cyclo-oxygenase and reduces prostaglandin production. Studies with indoprofen, *in vitro*, have demonstrated that it reduces PMN migration and their release of prostaglandins.

Single-dose studies in normal volunteers and patients with rheumatoid arthritis have shown that it is rapidly absorbed when taken orally and that peak concentrations are achieved within two hours. Indoprofen is strongly bound to plasma proteins and has an elimination half-life of about two hours. It is distributed readily to the synovial fluid. Most of the drug is eliminated renally, following extensive metabolism to the glucuronide.

Indoprofen is used in patients with rheumatoid arthritis, osteoarthritis, acute gout and soft-tissue rheumatism. It has also been given intra-articularly to patients with rheumatoid arthritis and used as an analgesic agent in patients with post-operative pain and secondary carcinoma. Clinical trials have shown it to be useful as an anti-inflammatory analgesic agent, with a similar spectrum of side-effects to other NSAIDs, the adverse reactions reported most frequently being gastro-intestinal. Skin rashes and neurological side-effects may sometimes occur. Indoprofen has no significant effects on renal function over a one-month treatment period in patients with rheumatoid arthritis. No significant interactions have been reported with oral hypoglycaemic agents, frusemide or warfarin.

Indoprofen is available in 100 mg and 200 mg capsules and as intramuscular, intra-articular or intravenous preparations. Although it has a short half-life, its efficacy in rheumatoid arthritis has been demonstrated with a twice-daily regimen.

Suprofen

Suprofen is an acetic acid derivative, *RS*-α + methyl-4-(2-thienylcarbonyl) benzene acetic acid (figure 5.12). It has been shown to have analgesic, anti-pyretic and anti-inflammatory effects in animal models and, like other NSAIDs, interferes with prostaglandin production. It is rapidly absorbed from the gastro-intestinal tract and reaches peak plasma concentrations after one hour. Metabolism is primarily by ester glucuronidation followed by renal elimination. Suprofen is strongly bound to plasma proteins. Clinically it has been used in analgesic studies. At a dose of 200 mg it is as effective an analgesic as 650 mg

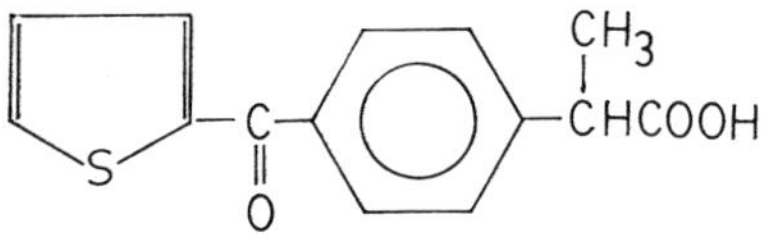

Figure 5.12. Suprofen.

aspirin plus 60 mg of codeine. The duration of analgesia is approximately four to six hours and correlates with peak plasma concentrations. It is effective in a variety of conditions including dysmenorrhoea, post-partum pain, episiotomy and dental pain and a variety of soft-tissue musculoskeletal, conditions.

Further studies are required before the relative efficacy of suprofen as an NSAID can be assessed. Currently, its use would be as an analgesic in doses of 200 mg three or four times daily.

Tiaprofen

Tiaprofenic acid, *RS*-5-benzoyl-α-methyl-2-thiophene acetic acid, (figure 5.13) has been shown to have analgesic, anti-pyretic and anti-inflammatory activities in classic animal models of inflammation. It inhibits cyclo-oxygenase, but has little effect on the lipoxygenase system.

Pharmacokinetic studies in normal volunteers have shown rapid absorption after oral administration, with peak plasma concentrations being reached within one hour. The drug is rapidly metabolized to compounds which are less active than the parent. Urinary excretion in man accounts for approximately 60% of the oral dose and serial studies have failed to show any inhibition or induction of metabolism with time. Tiaprofenic acid has a short elimination half-life and is strongly bound to plasma protein. The drug diffuses rapidly into synovial fluid, and four hours after administration, synovial fluid concentrations slightly exceed those seen in the plasma.

Tiaprofenic acid is used in the treatment of osteoarthritis and rheumatoid arthritis. Doses between 600 and 1200 mg per day are effective, but doses of 1200 mg are associated with an increase in liver enzymes. Adverse reactions reported with tiaprofenic acid are similar to other NSAIDs, with gastro-intestinal side-effects being most common. Bioavailability of tiaprofenic acid is not influenced by aluminium hydroxide, salicylates or phenprocoumon.

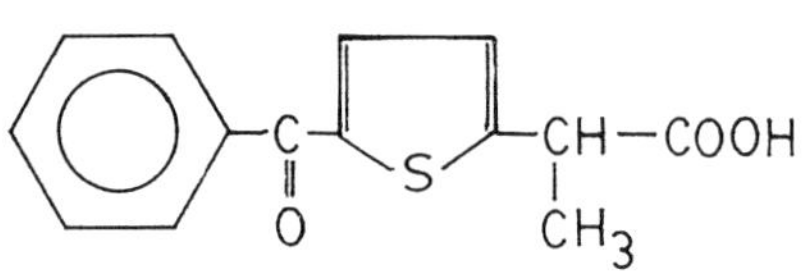

Figure 5.13. Tiaprofen.

Furthermore, tiaprofenic acid does not affect prothrombin time in patients taking phenprocoumon.

Tiaprofenic acid in doses of between 600 and 1200 mg daily can be useful in the treatment of osteoarthritis and rheumatoid arthritis, although further studies are required before its comparative efficacy with other NSAIDs can be assessed.

Fenbufen

Fenbufen, γ-oxo(1,1-biphenyl)-4-butanoic acid, (figure 5.14) is soluble in alkaline solution and has been shown to have analgesic, anti-pyretic and anti-inflammatory activity. Anti-inflammatory activity is found in both the parent compound and its major metabolite, biphenylacetic acid, although prostaglandin synthetase is inhibited by the metabolite only, suggesting that metabolism is required for anti-inflammatory effect.

Following oral administration fenbufen is rapidly absorbed, peak plasma concentrations being achieved within two hours. Absorption is delayed, but not significantly decreased when fenbufen is administered with food. The drug is extensively metabolized in man and excreted in the urine. At least two metabolites (biphenylacetic and γ-hydroxybiphenylbutanoic acid) are active in man. Fenbufen is strongly bound to plasma proteins, distributed to the synovial fluid and found in low concentrations in breast milk. The elimination half-life is about 10 hours in patients with rheumatoid arthritis given a single 600 mg dose. There is no evidence of drug toxicity in patients with renal impairment, but the concentrations of some metabolites increase, while others decrease.

Fenbufen has been shown to be effective against rheumatoid arthritis, osteoarthritis, gout, and non-articular rheumatism. In studies it has been shown to be better than placebo, but no better than comparative NSAIDs. It is well tolerated in the majority of patients with rheumatoid arthritis or osteoarthritis. The major side-effects are gastro-intestinal, leading to withdrawal of therapy in approximately 4% of patients. CNS effects such as headache and dizziness occur infrequently with fenbufen compared to indomethacin, and mild skin rashes occur in approximately 5% of patients. Liver enzymes are occasionally elevated.

Concurrent aspirin therapy reduces plasma drug concentrations following a single dose, but the clinical effect of this interaction is unknown. Concurrent

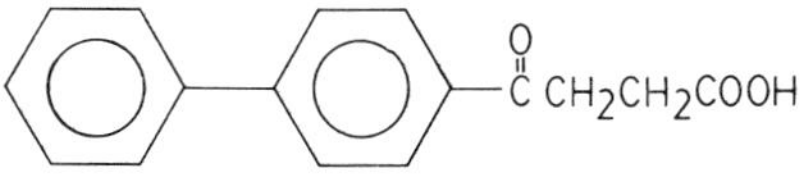

Figure 5.14. Fenbufen.

administration with digoxin results in a slight increase in digoxin serum concentration, but this is thought to be clinically irrelevant. In ten healthy subjects given fenbufen, there was a significant decrease in mean daily plasma warfarin concentration, but the clinical relevance of this is unclear. Antacid administration does not affect the bioavailability of fenbufen.

Fenbufen is available in 100 and 200 mg tablets and the usual dose is 600–1000 mg/day. It is usually administered twice daily, but there is some evidence that a single dose, taken at night, may be as effective in a proportion of patients with arthritis.

Diflunisal

Diflunisal is a derivative of salicylic acid, but has no O-acetyl group and therefore does not participate in protein acetylation. The structure of diflunisal and acetylsalicylic acid are shown in figure 5.15.

Diflunisal has been shown to have analgesic, anti-pyretic and anti-inflammatory effects in animal models and its mechanism of action relies on the inhibition of cyclo-oxygenase. It has a reversible effect on platelet function and significant uricosuric activity. In studies on a variety of laboratory models no increased foetal death rate, effect on reproduction or fertility, or teratogenic effects were observed.

Diflunisal is rapidly absorbed after oral administration with peak plasma concentrations found within two hours of oral administration. Food reduces the peak plasma concentration, but does not alter bioavailability. Diflunisal is strongly bound to plasma proteins, but has a low volume of distribution. It is almost completely excreted in the urine, appearing as soluble glucuronide conjugates. The elimination half-life varies with dose, from five hours with 50 mg to 15 hours following a single 1 g dose. Elimination is dependent on renal function, but marked prolongation of plasma half-life does not occur until creatinine clearance falls below 30 ml/min. Alkalinization of urine has been used to enhance urinary excretion.

Diflunisal was introduced initially as an analgesic agent, but it has potent anti-inflammatory activities too. It is useful in the treatment of osteoarthritis,

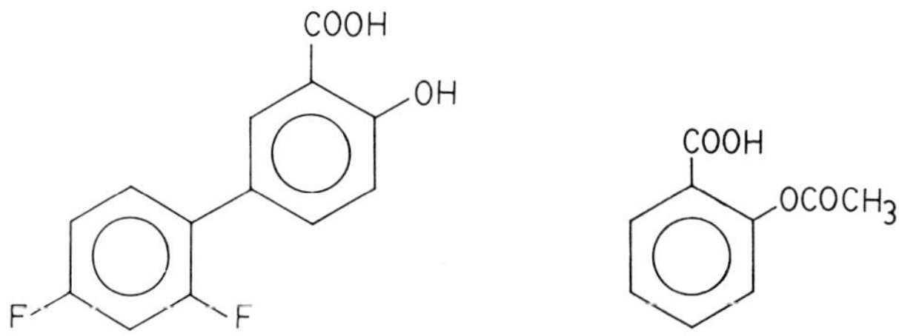

Figure 5.15. Diflunisal and acetylsalicylic acid.

rheumatoid arthritis, and a variety of painful conditions including post-traumatic pain, dental pain and pain due to malignant disease. Single-dose analgesic studies employ between 250 and 500 mg, while daily doses of 500–1000 mg/day have been used in osteoarthritis and rheumatoid arthritis. Diflunisal producces fewer gastro-intestinal side-effects than aspirin and does not cause ototoxicity. Absorption is reduced by the concomitant administration of aluminium hydroxide, but magnesium hydroxide does not affect bioavailability. Bioavailability is reduced by the administration of aspirin. Although the percentage of unbound warfarin is increased by concomitant diflunisal treatment, no significant effect on anti-coagulation is seen. This interaction is complex, however, as, on discontinuation of diflunisal, the anti-coagulant effect of warfarin is reduced, although the total concentration remains unchanged. There is no interaction between tolbutamide and diflunisal, but co-administration of diflunisal with indomethacin results in an increase in plasma indomethacin concentration, together with a decreased indomethacin renal clearance. Diflunisal has been shown to counteract the hyperuricaemic effect of thiazide diuretics and to increase their plasma concentrations.

Diflunisal is available in 250 mg and 500 mg tablets and the usual daily dose is between 500 and 1000 mg. Diflunisal is contra-indicated in patients who are hypersensitive to aspirin, or who have previously experienced episodes of bronchospasm precipitated by aspirin or other NSAIDs.

Fenamates

The fenamates are N-arylanthranilic acids which have been used as NSAIDs for a number of years. The structures of the currently used fenamates, flufenamic acid, mefenamic acid and meclofenamic acid are shown in figure 5.16.

All have analgesic, anti-pyretic and anti-inflammatory effects in animal models of inflammation and inhibit prostaglandin-synthetase activity.

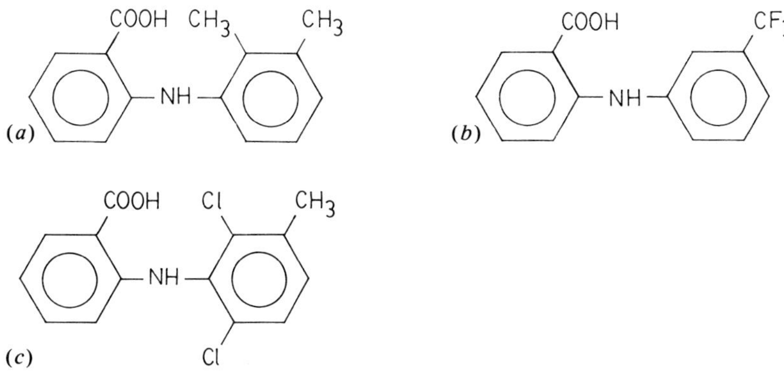

Figure 5.16. The fenamates; (*a*) mefenamic acid, (*b*) flufenamic acid and (*c*) meclofenamic acid.

Meclofenamic acid may inhibit lipoxygenase activity also, causing the decreased synthesis of leukotrienes.

Mefenamic acid is rapidly absorbed after oral administration with peak plasma concentrations occuring within about two hours. Flufenamic acid is absorbed more slowly with peak concentrations occurring in about six hours. Both have relatively short half-lives with approximately 50% being recovered in the urine as either unchanged drug or as oxidized or hydroxylated metabolites. In addition, the fenamates undergo considerable biliary recycling, which results in prolonged retention in the body. Like other acidic NSAIDs, they are strongly bound to plasma proteins.

Flufenamic acid and mefenamic acid have been shown to be superior to a placebo in the treatment of rheumatoid arthritis, osteoarthritis and soft-tissue rheumatism. Although beneficial in inflammatory joint disease, their use has not been widespread owing to the relatively high incidence of diarrhoea. Dyspepsia also occurs with these agents, but its incidence is similar to that seen with other NSAIDs. Maculo-papular rashes have been reported with both flufenamic and mefenamic acid, but these subside rapidly on withdrawal of the drug. Mefenamic acid has been used extensively for the treatment of dysmenorrhoea and, in this situation, the short duration of treatment is not associated with significant side-effects.

Meclofenamic acid has recently been introduced as an effective treatment for rheumatoid arthritis, osteoarthritis, acute gout, ankylosing spondylitis and post-traumatic oedema. The major side-effects are again seen in the gastro-intestinal tract, with indigestion and diarrhoea being most common. Meclofenamic acid would seem to be a useful alternative to other NSAIDs, with a similar spectrum of activity and side-effects, apart from a slightly increased risk of diarrhoea.

Mefenamic acid is marketed in 250 mg tablets with the recommended daily dose being 1 to 1.5 g. Flufenamic acid is marketed as 100 mg or 200 mg capsules and its recommended daily dose is 400 to 600 mg. Meclofenamic acid is available in 100 mg capsules with a recommended daily dose of 200 to 400 mg for rheumatoid arthritis and osteoarthritis, a higher initial dose being used in the short-term for the treatment of acute gout.

Oxicams

The oxicams piroxicam, isoxicam and sudoxicam belong to a series of N-heterocyclic carboxamides of 1,2-benzothiazine-1,1-dioxide (see figure 5.17).

Piroxicam

Piroxicam was the first of the oxicams to be introduced into clinical practice and has analgesic, anti-pyretic and anti-inflammatory activity. It stabilizes lysosomal membranes, but inhibits the secondary phase of platelet aggre-

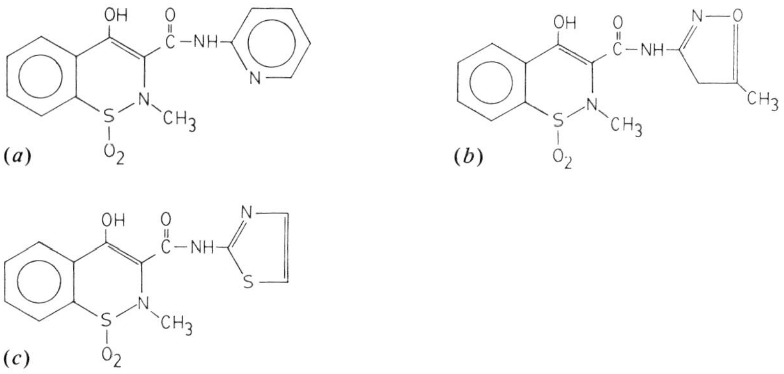

Figure 5.17. The oxicams, (*a*) piroxicam, (*b*) isoxicam and (*c*) sudoxicam.

gation, induced by adenosine diphosphate, as well as prostaglandin synthesis, the chemotaxis of PMNs and phagocytosis. Extensive toxicological studies have failed to demonstrate any affect on embryo viability or foetal body weight in rats and rabbits, but like other NSAIDs it induces gastro-intestinal lesions and renal papillary necrosis in rats and dogs treated with piroxicam for 12 to 18 months.

Piroxicam is rapidly absorbed following oral or rectal administration with peak plasma concentrations being obtained two hours after oral, and six hours after rectal administration. Mean steady-state plasma concentrations are achieved after seven days. The plasma elimination half-life of piroxicam, in normal subjects, is about 38 hours and does not seem to be related to dose. There is considerable variation in plasma half-life between normal individuals (14–160 hours). At therapeutic concentrations plasma-protein binding is in excess of 99%. Piroxicam accumulates in the synovial fluid, where the synovial fluid to plasma ratio is approximately 0.4 to 1.

Piroxicam is extensively metabolized in man and there is some evidence of entero-hepatic recycling. The principal metabolite, produced by hydroxylation and then conjugated with glucuronic acid, is at least 1000 times less active than piroxicam in inhibiting cyclo-oxygenase activity.

Steady-state plasma drug concentrations do not seem to be affected by food, concomitant ferrous sulphate therapy, or concurrent antacids containing aluminium hydroxide alone or in combination with magnesium hydroxide. Although changes may occur with concomitant aspirin therapy there is no evidence of a clinically significant interaction.

Piroxicam has been shown to be effective in the treatment of rheumatoid arthritis, osteoarthritis, acute gout, ankylosing spondylitis, and soft-tissue rheumatism. Most studies have been conducted at a dose of 20 mg/day and have shown clear differences between drug and placebo as well as a similar efficacy to other NSAIDs. The minimum effective dose of piroxicam has not been determined, although it is possible that doses of 10 mg per day may be effective for many patients with inflammatory joint disease. The advantages of this drug are that steady-state plasma concentrations can be achieved with a single daily dose, and it has a relatively low incidence of side-effects. The side-effects seen are those common to other NSAIDs, gastro-intestinal complaints being most frequent. Headache, dizziness, skin rashes and ankle oedema are rare. Transient elevations of liver enzymes or blood urea have been reported also. No significant changes in glomerular-filtration rate were noted during the treatment of a small number of patients with osteoarthritis.

Piroxicam is available in 10 mg tablets and most patients can be controlled on a dose of between 10 and 20 mg/day. Some patients will require higher doses, but these are associated with an increased risk of gastro-intestinal side-effects. To treat acute gout 40 mg of piroxicam should be given daily for 4 to 6 days, then the dose reduced to 10 to 20 mg/day.

Isoxicam

Isoxicam is the newest of the oxicam derivatives to be introduced. It is poorly soluble in water (2μg/ml) and has a pK_a of 3.6. The drug is anti-pyretic, analgesic and anti-inflammatory in standard animal test sytems, its mechanism of action probably being due to suppression of cyclo-oxygenase.

Isoxicam is readily absorbed following oral administration with peak plasma concentrations being achieved within four to eight hours. The oral bioavailability of about 70%, in fasting subjects, is increased when isoxicam is given with food. It is strongly bound to plasma proteins (95 to 98%) and displays linear pharmacokinetics over a 100–400 mg dose range. Isoxicam is extensively metabolized in man, with less than 2% of the dose excreted unchanged in the urine. Its metabolism occurs primarily by hydroxymethylation and since it has a low total-body clearance there is a long elimination half-life of approximately 31 hours. There is marked individual variation in this prolonged half-life, but steady-state plasma concentrations are generally achieved within 12 days.

Isoxicam has been used in the treatment of rheumatoid- and osteo-arthritis where it has significant anti-inflammatory and analgesic activity. Although the spectrum of side-effects is similar to that of other NSAIDs there have been a number of recent reports of Stevens-Johnson syndrome and toxic epidermal necrolysis. Following reports of fatalities due to these skin conditions in patients receiving isoxicam, the drug has been placed under review and is not currently being marketed. Concurrent administration of aspirin produces lower plasma isoxicam concentrations, the clinical significance of which is uncertain. Isoxicam increases the anti-coagulant effects of warfarin, but does not interact with cimetidine.

Isoxicam was available in 100 mg tablets and the standard daily dose was between 100 and 300 mg.

Pyrazole derivatives

The original pyrazoles, phenylbutazone and its metabolite oxyphenbutazone, have been available for over 30 years. Recently two new derivatives azapropazone and feprazone have been described.

Phenylbutazone and oxyphenbutazone

The chemical structures of phenylbutazone and its major metabolite hydroxyphenylbutazone (oxyphenbutazone) are shown in figure 5.18. Phenylbutazone was the first of the NSAIDs to be introduced in the 1950s. It has analgesic, anti-pyretic and anti-inflammatory effects in animal models and mediates these effects by inhibiting cyclo-oxygenase, stabilizing lysosomal membranes and proteins and interfering with platelet aggregation.

Following oral administration, phenylbutazone is rapidly and completely absorbed from the small intestine. Peak plasma concentrations are reached within four hours and the drug elimination half-life attained in 72 hours. Oxyphenbutazone has a slightly shorter half-life, but both drugs are extensively bound to plasma proteins and have relatively small volumes of distribution. Phenylbutazone is extensively metabolized in man and only about 1% of the administered dose is excreted unchanged in the urine. Enterohepatic circulation of the metabolite dihydroxyphenylbutazone occurs in man, and phenylbutazone exhibits both dose- and time-dependent pharmacokinetics. Although clinical trials demonstrate the efficacy of both phenylbutazone and oxyphenbutazone in rheumatoid arthritis, sero-negative spondyloarthropathies, gout, osteoarthritis and a variety of other rheumatic conditions, the incidence of fatal adverse reactions has led to a recent re-appraisal of their prescription. Over the last 20 years at least 1000 persons have died from aplastic anaemic or neutropaenia associated with use of phenylbutazone or oxyphenbutazone. Owing to the availability of other NSAIDs, its use should, therefore, be reserved for those patients with ankylosing spondylitis, or a sero-negative arthropathy not responding to indomethacin or a propionic-acid derivative, patients with rheumatoid arthritis who do not respond to other NSAIDs and patients with acute gouty arthritis failing to respond to indomethacin and colchicine. Phenylbutazone and oxyphenbutazone should not be used in the treatment of osteoarthritis or soft-tissue rheumatism.

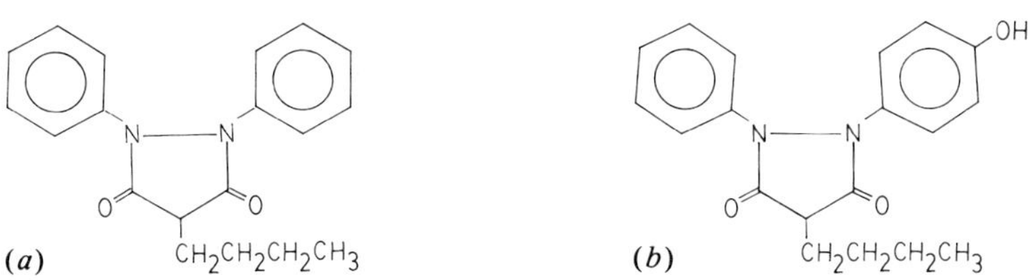

Figure 5.18. (*a*) Phenylbutazone and (*b*) oxyphenbutazone.

Significant interactions occur between phenylbutazone and coumarin anti-coagulants enhancing the anti-coagulant response. The enhancement is caused by the inhibition of metabolism of the *S* enantiomer of warfarin. Phenylbutazone and oxyphenbutazone also interfere with the metabolism of the sulphonylurea, oral hypoglycaemic agents, producing hypoglycaemia.

Phenylbutazone is available in 100 and 200 mg tablets either plain or enteric coated, and as a suppository. A 100 mg tablet combined with aluminium hydroxide and magnesium trisilicate is also available, but it is not clear whether this effectively reduces the incidence of gastric irritation. An intra-muscular preparation is provided, but as this is irritant its use is not recommended.

Azapropazone

Azapropazone, 5-dimethylamino-9-methyl-2-propyl-1H-pyrazolo-(1,2-α)(1,2,4)-benzotriazine-1,3(2H)-dione dihydrate, has some structural similarities to phenylbutazone (figure 5.19). Like other NSAIDs it is very slightly soluble in water.

It has analgesic, anti-pyretic and anti-inflammatory effects in animal models. Azapropazone is rapidly absorbed from the gastro-intestinal tract following oral administration with peak plasma concentrations being seen within four hours. The drug is strongly bound to plasma proteins and so the apparent volume of distribution is relatively low (0.1 to 0.15 l/kg). The plasma elimination half-life of azapropazone is about 12 hours and most of the drug is excreted in the urine unchanged. Plateau plasma concentrations are reached after five days of repeated administration. Azapropazone readily enters synovial fluid, but peak concentrations are delayed, being seen 24 hours after an oral dose. Doses should be reduced in those with renal or hepatic dysfunction since these patients have reduced plasma clearance.

Azapropazone is effective in the treatment of rheumatoid arthritis, osteo-arthritis, ankylosing spondylitis, gout, and soft-tissue rheumatism. Doses between 900 and 1200 mg/day are used. The use of azapropazone in acute gout is particularly important as it significantly reduces the concentration of

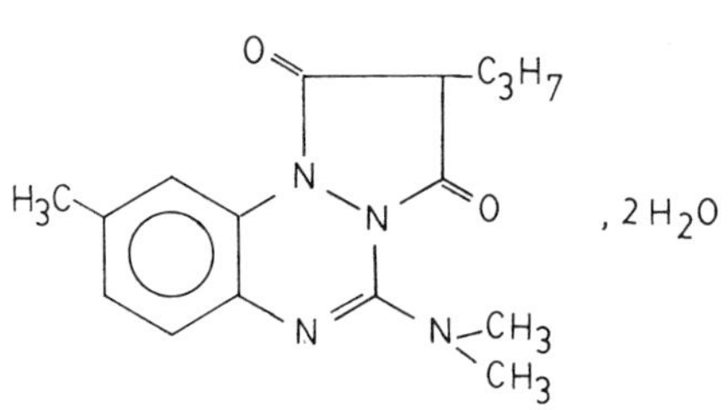

Figure 5.19. Azapropazone.

uric acid in the serum. The side-effects of azapropazone are those noted with other NSAIDs, gastric intolerance being the most common. Although it is structurally related to phenylbutazone there are no reports of serious bone marrow toxicity.

Azapropazone displaces warfarin from human serum albumin and significantly increases phenytoin plasma levels. It is available in capsule form (300 mg) or as a film-coated tablet (600 mg). The total daily dose required varies from 600 to 1200 mg, except in acute gout where 2.4 g/day may be required initially. Azapropazone can be administered twice daily, although a single dose may provide adequate symptomatic relief in many patients.

Choice of non-steroidal anti-inflammatory drug

It seems clear that there is considerable variation in response to NSAIDs in terms of both pain relief and adverse drug reactions. The reasons for this are not clear and studies in this area have been difficult to interpret because of a failure to measure the active drug or metabolite in the synovial fluid or tissue. Many NSAIDs exist as *S*- and *R*- enantiomers. The *S*-enantiomer is the active anti-inflammatory form of the propionic-acid derivatives, but while naproxen is administered entirely as the *S*-enantiomer, other NSAIDs are administered as racemates and undergo conversion *in vivo*. It is possible that individuals convert the enantiomers at different rates and this could explain some of the variability in response.

Although many NSAIDs have a relatively short plasma half-life their duration of action in terms of pain relief seems much longer. There is increasing evidence that drugs with short half-lives (e.g. ibuprofen, flurbiprofen, diclofenac) can be given less frequently than would be predicted by their plasma concentrations. Pharmacokinetic studies have shown that NSAIDs collect in the synovial fluid where they may be sustained for longer periods of time than in the plasma. There is also evidence that the inhibition of cyclo-oxygenase continues for some time after they have disappeared from the synovial fluid. This suggests that NSAIDs may be given less frequently without any significant reduction in anti-inflammatory effect.

Side-effects vary with individuals. Indigestion is particularly common but is more likely to occur with drugs such as aspirin or indomethacin than with propionic-acid derivatives. However, marked individual susceptibility occurs and if one agent causes indigestion then it should be stopped and another one tried. It is unusual to find patients unable to tolerate any NSAID because of indigestion. Many NSAIDs cause fluid retention, particularly in the elderly, and the prescribing physician should be aware of this complication. They may also interfere with the action of anti-hypertensive agents, particularly beta-adrenergic blocking drugs, or diuretics. Acute renal failure has been described in association with a number of NSAIDs and many patients demonstrate a transient decrease in renal function: in most situations renal function returns to normal despite continuation of the NSAID but care should be taken in patients who have underlying renal disease, chronic hepatic disease, congestive cardiac failure, sodium depletion or who are on long-term diuretic therapy. It is likely that these side-effects may be more prolonged in patients prescribed NSAIDs with long half-lives. Pro-drugs such as sulindac may have less effect on renal function and these should be considered in patients who are at risk.

The development of new NSAIDs has meant that patients do not need to take large quantities of salicylates to suppress pain and inflammation. NSAIDs can be given one or twice a day despite their short plasma half-life, although efficacy can sometimes be prolonged by the use of slow-release formulations. Enteric-coated or slow-release formulations will also reduce gastric irritation and in situations where this persists the drug may be given by suppository.

Certain rheumatic diseases seem to respond better to some NSAIDs than to others. This is particularly so for the seronegative spondyloarthropathies which often show little response to salicylates, but improve significantly when treated with indomethacin. Most NSAIDs seem to be effective in the treatment of rheumatoid arthritis whereas the propionic-acid derivatives and diclofenac can be used for osteoarthritis and soft-tissue rheumatism. As patients with arthritis, in particular rheumatoid arthritis, have morning stiffness, the largest proportion of the daily dose should be given at night or a sustained-release preparation used.

Although it is important to avoid drugs in pregnancy it is sometimes necessary to prescribe NSAIDs. All NSAIDs have the ability to prolong gestation and labour because of their effect on prostaglandin production. Some NSAIDs have been associated with an increased risk of anti- and post-partum haemorrhage and with the induction of pulmonary hypertension in the neonate. Thus, if they are required in pregnancy it is wise to use those drugs with short half-lives, such as the propionic-acid derivatives of diclofenac. The NSAIDs are also likely to be distributed to human breast milk and if prescribed during lactation NSAIDs with short half-lives and inactive metabolites such as propionic-acid derivatives or diclofenac should be used.

The optimal number of NSAIDs has not been determined, but there is little doubt that a range of drugs is required to allow patients to find the drug that suits them best in terms of pain relief and lack of side-effects. The choice of NSAID in a particular situation must remain an individual one but factors such as those shown in table 5.1 must be considered both for the drug and for the patient. Patients will respond to an NSAID within 10 to 14 days, at least in terms of pain relief, and the dose should be increased fairly quickly to the maximum tolerated dose. If the patient is not responding or develops a side-effect then the NSAID should be discontinued and an alternative started. Once a patient is well controlled continuing review of the disease should be undertaken. In many situations the dose and/or frequency of dosing may be reduced and, in situations such as osteoarthritis or soft-tissue rheumatism, the drug withdrawn completely.

Table 5.1. Factors to be considered when choosing a NSAID

In the patient	**In the drug**
Disease type and activity	Spectrum of side-effects
Age	Safety
Concomitant medications	Formulation
Other diseases	Dose and frequency of administration
	Pharmacokinetics
	Cost
	Compliance

NSAIDs provide symptomatic relief for patients with a wide variety of rheumatic complaints. Used carefully they can provide significant pain relief and reduce disability, although they must be used in conjunction with other forms of treatment, such as suppressive agents, physical treatments and educational strategies.

Further reading

Bonta, I. L., Parnham, M. J. Vincent, J. E. and Bragt, P. C., 1980, Anti-rheumatic drugs: Present deadlocks and new vistas. *Progress in Medicinal Chemistry*, **17**, 186–273.

Brooks, P. M. and Day, R. O. (editors), 1985, Non-steroidal anti-inflammatory drugs — basis for variability in response. (Birkhauser-Verlag, Basel).

Clinics in the Rheumatic Diseases: *Anti-Rheumatic Drugs*, 1979, 5(1), 351–736.

Clinics in the Rheumatic Diseases: *Anti-Rheumatic Drugs*, 1980, 6(2), 463–698.

Clinics in the Rheumatic Diseases: *Anti-Rheumatic Drugs*, 1984, 11(1), 219–432.

Hart, F. D. (editor), 1978, *Drug Treatment of the Rheumatic Diseases*, Adis Press, Auckland, New Zealand.

Editorial, 1984, Non-steroidal anti-inflammatory drugs: have we been spoilt for choice? *Lancet*, **1**, 141.

Graham, G. G., Day, R. O., Champion, G. D., Lee, E. and Newton, K., 1984, Aspects of the clinical pharmacology of non-steroidal anti-inflammatory drugs. *Clinics in the Rheumatic Diseases*, **10**, 229–249.

Huskisson, E. C., 1984, How to choose a non-steroidal anti-inflammatory drug. *Clinics in the Rheumatic Diseases*, **10**, 313–323.

Needs, C. J. and Brooks, P. M. 1985, Occasional reviews: Anti-rheumatic drugs in pregnancy. Anti-rheumatic drugs during lactation. *British Journal of Rheumatology*, **24**, 282–297.

Veerbeeck, R. K., Blackburn, J. J. and Loewen, G. R. 1983, Clinical pharmacokinetics of non-steroidal anti-inflammatory drugs. *Clinical Pharmacokinetics*, **8**, 297–331.

6. Slow-acting anti-rheumatic drugs

Anti-malarials

Chloroquine phosphate and hydroxychloroquine sulphate

Chloroquine phosphate and hydroxychloroquine sulphate are 4-amino-7-chloroquinoline compounds. The 4-aminoquinolines were synthesized during the early part of this century, and were used during World War II as a treatment for malaria. Subsequently, it was recognized that chloroquine and hydroxychloroquine were of value in the treatment of rheumatoid disease, systemic lupus, discoid lupus and other connective-tissue diseases. Chloroquine diphosphate is a white bitter powder which is soluble in water. The D-isomer is less toxic than the L-isomer. Chloroquine differs from hydroxychloroquine in that the *N*-ethyl portion of chloroquine is β-hydroxylated, otherwise the structure is equivalent to the parent molecule (figure 6.1). Chloroquine phosphate is available as 250 and 500 mg tablets and can be given by injection as the chloroquine hydrochloride which is available in 5 ml ampoules, each containing 50 mg/ml. Hydroxychloroquine sulphate is available in 200 mg tablets equivalent to 250 mg of base. Thus, 400 mg of hydroxychloroquine sulphate is equivalent to 500 mg of chloroquine phosphate.

Mechanisms of action

Like other agents used to treat rheumatoid arthritis, the definitive mechanism of action of the 4-aminoquinolines has not been determined. Chloroquine and hydroxychloroquine do not exhibit any noticeable clinical effect until they have been used for 8 to 12 weeks. It is, therefore, particularly interesting that chloroquine has been shown to interfere with sulphydryl–disulphide exchange, an action common to the injectable gold complexes and D-penicillamine. In the serum concentrations found in rheumatoid patients, chloroquine inhibits the reduction of ferricyanide by cysteine and binds to proteins containing SH groups. The capacity of chloroquine and hydroxychloroquine to react with SH groups makes these drugs capable of interacting with pleuropneumonia-like organisms and most viruses.

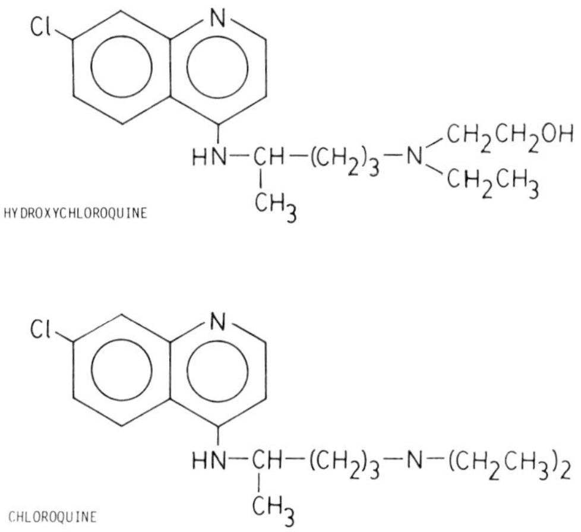

Figure 6.1. The anti-malarials.

Anti-malarial drugs exhibit several effects on the inflammatory response. Mepacrine can suppress prostaglandin activity by exerting a direct effect on phospholipase A2, but the most significant effect demonstrated by anti-malarials *in vivo* is a direct antagonism of prostaglandin production by chloroquine and it is thought that this occurs through membrane binding or alteration of prostaglandin membrane binding sites. Chloroquine also competes with prostaglandins for DNA binding and suppresses DNA and RNA synthesis. The anti-malarials inhibit the action of lysosomal enzymes such as neutral protease and collagenase and also stabilize lysosomal membranes. PMN migration, phagocytosis and chemotaxis are inhibited by chloroquine. It is difficult to relate some of these *in-vitro* and *in-vivo* studies to the definitive action in patients, since the concentrations were 100–1000 times greater than those used therapeutically.

One other *in-vitro* mechanism of the anti-malarials, which resembles the action of injectable gold compounds, is the inhibition of lymphocyte responsiveness to mitogens. Recently, it has been shown that chloroquine, in therapeutic concentration, inhibits lymphocyte responsiveness by selectively blocking the release of interleukin-1 from monocytes.

Although no definitive mechanism has been determined for the action of the anti-malarials in the treatment of rheumatoid disease, systemic lupus and discoid lupus, the similarity of certain mechanisms to those of gold compounds, D-penicillamine and some immuno-suppressives points to a common therapeutic action or actions. This is further supported by the fact that the clinical response to chloroquine in rheumatoid disease occurs 10 to 12 weeks after the start of treatment, a time span similar to that observed with injectable gold compounds and D-penicillamine.

Pharmacokinetics

Following oral ingestion both chloroquine and hydroxychloroquine are rapidly and completely absorbed from the gastro-intestinal tract. Approximately 50–55% of either compound is protein bound and the rest remains in equilibrium with the tissue. With a dose of 300 mg of chloroquine base per day, serum levels of 0.6 to 0.9 μmol/l are achieved, and for a daily dose of hydroxychloroquine of 400 mg/day, serum levels of 1.4 to 1.5 μmol/l are achieved. Owing to rapid absorption peak plasma concentrations are usually seen within the first 2 to 10 hours. Both drugs are extensively distributed in the tissues in various concentrations: up to 1×10^{-3} M being found in melanized tissue; 3×10^{-4} M in the liver, spleen and white cells; and 4×10^{-6} M in red blood cells, muscle and brain. The concentration in fat, bone and tendon is considerably lower, 1×10^{-6} M. It is this avidity for melanized tissue which accounts for the retinopathy associated with the chloroquine compounds. The metabolism of hydroxychloroquine differs from chloroquine in that the former produces two first-stage metabolites of the desethylhydroxychloroquine type. Following the degradation of chloroquine, approximately 25% appears as desethylchloroquine in the urine. Metabolism further proceeds to the bis-desethyl derivatives of both chloroquine and hydroxychloroquine and, subsequently, to the 4′-aldehyde and 4′-carboxy derivatives. Approximately 60–70% of the drug is excreted in the urine with approximately 10% of chloroquine and up to 20% of hydroxychloroquine being found in the faeces. Hydroxychloroquine is also conjugated with the glucuronide and undergoes biliary excretion. Approximately 50–70% of the urinary product is unchanged drug; 10–25% is a monodesethylchloroquine and 2% bis-desethylchloroquine. The elimination half-life of both chloroquine and hydroxychloroquine appears to be multi-phasic. The pharmacokinetics of the anti-malarials is complex and may be non-linear, such that more than proportional accumulation of parent drug or metabolite occurs. The anti-malarials have a large volume of distribution due to avid tissue-binding characteristics. The multi-phasic half-life is related to a small plasma component and a large cellular component. The cellular component comprises parenchymal cells from the liver, spleen, marrow, muscle and skin as well as leucocytes. Approximately 50% of the drug is bound to the nucleus and 50% is contained in the lysosomes. The cytoplasm and microsomal structures generally do not contain any drug. The avidity of chloroquine and hydroxychloroquine for melanin tissues is so great that these drugs may be detected years after drug therapy has been discontinued.

Clinical use of anti-malarials

The indication for starting a patient on anti-malarials is exactly the same as for gold and D-penicillamine, namely failure of the patient to respond to a careful, unhurried trial of NSAIDs. They are also useful in the treatment of systemic lupus erythematosus, particularly in those patients who have experienced a skin rash, and in discoid lupus. The recommended dosage is 250 mg/day of chloroquine phosphate and 200 mg/day of hydroxychloroquine sulphate and patients should be advised to take their tablets with food. Owing to the potential for eye toxicity, a routine ophthalmological examination should be carried out before therapy is instituted. Approximately 75% of patients will gain benefit from the use of these compounds, but a small portion of approximately 10% will have a significantly high degree of disease suppression. The percentage of patients who withdraw from drug therapy due to side-effects is generally around 10%.

Double-blind controlled trials in the 1960s confirmed the preliminary observations made in the 1950s. Chloroquine was shown to be better than placebo and its clinical efficacy continues to improve up to and beyond two years of administration. Investigators found a reduction in the number of inflamed joints, and improvement in joint function, ESR, functional capacity and patient satisfaction and reduction in rheumatoid-factor titre. There is no evidence to date that chloroquine or hydroxychloroquine prevents the development or progression of bone erosions. In 1977, Dwosh and colleagues followed patients given myochrisine, chloroquine and azathioprine, for 24 weeks and found no significant differences among the three drugs. However, chloroquine was slightly less effective than gold and azathioprine. To date there have been no double-blind controlled studies on the use of anti-malarial compounds in juvenile arthritis, or in their efficacy in elderly patients. MacKenzie and Sherbel recommend the use of anti-malarials in the treatment of Sjogren's syndrome, scleroderma, myositis and psoriatic arthropathy, but state that chloroquine does not appear to be beneficial in the treatment of ankylosing spondylitis or other HLA B27-associated diseases. To date there are no specific guidelines as to the duration of therapy, although disease suppression continues to be effective for up to four years.

Side-effects and contra-indications

Although low doses of the anti-malarials have been used safely during pregnancy for the treatment of malaria, we recommend that the drug be stopped in patients with rheumatoid disease or any other connective-tissue disease, if pregnancy occurs. However, while it was felt that psoriasis was a direct contra-indication to the use of anti-malarials, MacKenzie and Sherbel believe that this is no longer the case and that the development of erythroderma and exfoliative dermatitis is an allergic response, occuring in only 1 to 2% of patients. They state that patients are prepared to accept this small risk rather than take anti-metabolic drugs. Nevertheless, patients with a previous known allergic reaction to anti-malarials or with a family history of retinitis pigmentosa should not be given these compounds. Finally, patients with myasthenia gravis or any pre-existing myopathy should not receive chloroquine since this drug has been shown to depress muscle contractility.

The most common side-effects related to anti-malarial therapy are benign. Some 50–70% of patients will experience abdominal bloating, borborygmi and flatulence and approximately 30% of patients will develop diarrhoea. Nausea and vomiting after ingestion is uncommon, but for many patients the extremely bitter taste of the chloroquine tablet is unacceptable. Altered skin pigmentation can occur and bleaching or greying of the hair is experienced by patients exposed to high doses of ultraviolet light or excessive sunlight.

Eye toxicity

Fear of the development of eye toxicity, by both physician and patient, is the greatest limiting factor to the introduction of anti-malarial therapy for the treatment of rheumatoid disease, systemic lupus and discoid lupus. Retinopathy is the most dangerous effect of toxicity, but other side-effects occur. A cyclic ophthalmoplegia, resulting in a difficulty or delay in focusing, may develop shortly after starting chloroquine or hydroxychloroquine. Patients should be advised of this potential problem and the dosage reduced to 125 mg or 100 mg, for the chloroquine or hydroxychloroquine, respectively, until accommodation is normal. The cause of the ophthalmoplegia is thought to be the effect of the drugs on the muscle of the iris, and rarely, some patients may experience loss of the corneal reflex. This is a potentially dangerous situation and the dose should be reduced or stopped accordingly. Patients with dry eyes, secondary to Sjogren's syndrome, are at risk of developing corneal deposits of unchanged salts of chloroquine and hydroxychloroquine. Although these lesions are reversible and not related to retinopathy, the dosage should be reduced. Slit-lamp microscopic examination is the best means of detecting the lesions and should be carried out routinely, at the same time as the routine fundal examination.

The retina is a complex layer of neural tissue adapted for light reception and transmission, via the optic nerve, to the visual cortex. The cells that receive the light, the rods and cones, lie adjacent to the pigmented epithelium of the choroid. Some of the cells in this pigmented layer have macrophage-like functions and phagocytose the discarded photoreceptor membranes of the rods and cones. Chloroquine and hydroxychloroquine have a physical absorptive attraction for melanin and particles of melanin-bound chloroquine or hydroxychloroquine are engulfed by the pigmented epithelial cells. As stated above, the 4-aminoquinolines inhibit the release of lysosomal enzymes and decrease phagocytosis, chemotaxis and macrophage migration. The earliest indication of potential retinal toxicity is a reduction in the electrical potential generated by the pigmented epithelium. Increasing toxicity is indicated by night blindness and scotomata to red light. In more severe cases pigmented clumps or classical pigmented rings (Bull's-eye lesion) may be seen by fundoscopic examination. However, even at this stage, the majority of visual problems are reversible. With permanent visual damage, there are scotomata to white light, loss of visual acuity and Bull's-eye lesions. The retinal pigmentation associated with anti-malarial drug toxicity is similar to retinitis pigmentosa. Patients with this disease should not be given chloroquine or hydroxychloroquine, since these drugs may exacerbate the deficient metabolic properties of the pigmented epithelium. Retinal toxicity is rare provided adequate attention is paid to the drug dose and regular ophthalmological examinations are conducted every six months.

Drug–drug interactions

There are no known specific drug–drug interactions, but patients who develop a skin rash with gold compounds and/or D-penicillamine should be monitored carefully. It has been suggested that the concomitant use of hepatotoxic drugs or thioridazine be avoided, as these drugs have a similar spectrum of side-effects. Neither chloroquine or hydroxychloroquine should be administered during pregnancy.

Clinical guidelines

The majority of rheumatologists now use hydroxychloroquine in preference to chloroquine since it is believed that the former causes fewer side-effects. Hydroxychloroquine and an NSAID can be given to patients with inflammatory rheumatoid arthritis who have failed to respond to injectable gold compounds or to D-penicillamine. The starting dose of hydroxychloroquine should be 200 mg/day and this dose should be used throughout the course. A preliminary eye examination is essential and should be followed by a six-monthly review. It is wise to follow patients on hydroxychloroquine in a drug-monitoring clinic such as one used for patients receiving gold compounds or D-penicillamine. In such a setting, trained staff are on the look-out for subtle signs of toxicity. Benefit from the drug is usually observed after 8–12 weeks and continues for to 2 to 3 years. It is not known whether the long-term outcome of rheumatoid patients who receive hydroxychloroquine differs from that of patients who receive gold or D-penicillamine. Clinical trials indicate that during active disease anti-malarial drugs are better than placebo and only slightly less effective than gold or penicillamine.

Gold

Gold has been used for over 4000 years in the treatment of a wide variety of complaints, such as leprosy, syphilis and tuberculosis. However, it is only during the last 50 years that gold complexes have been applied to the treatment of rheumatic diseases.

Chemistry

Gold is classified as a Group 1B metal in the periodic table and has an electronic configuration of $[Xe]4f^{14}5d^{10}6s^1$. The most commonly recognized oxidation states are I, II, III and V (referred to in this text as Au(I) etc.), although metal–metal bonds may exist in complexes in which it is difficult to assign a formal oxidation state. Au(I) has a closed-shell electronic configuration, $[Xe]4f^{14}5d^{10}$, and thus, like the isoelectronic mercury (II), forms two, three and four-co-ordinate complexes. The Au(I) complexes are diamagnetic and adopt regular structures which are most commonly of the linear two-co-ordinate type. The true salts of Au(I), such as the halides, are unstable in the presence of water and disproportionate to Au^0 (metallic gold) and Au(III). However, Au(I) can be stabilized by the formation of complexes with 'soft' ligands, such as the thiolates and phosphines. All anti-arthritic gold complexes exist as Au(I) thiol or phosphine compounds. The Au(III) complexes are diamagnetic and have the low-spin $5d^8$ electron configuration. The vast majority of these then have a four co-ordinate square-planar stereochemistry. However, the high toxicity of Au(III) complexes, such as chloroauric acid ($HAuCl_4$), makes them unsuitable for human use. If gold sodium thiomalate is administered to laboratory animals, the gold recovered from the tissue and urine exists in the Au(I) oxidation state (i.e., the same oxidation state as the gold in gold sodium thiomalate) and not in the Au(III) oxidation state. Furthermore, if $Au(III)Cl_3$ is administered to laboratory animals, the gold recovered in tissues and urine exists only in the Au(I) oxidation state as determined by X-ray absorption near-edge spectroscopy (XANES) and extended X-ray absorption fine-structure spectroscopy (EXAFS). XANES can distinguish the Au(III) complex from Au(I) and Au^0 since it alone has a transition. EXAFS, with appropriate curve-fitting techniques, demonstrates that the gold atoms in a solution of gold sodium thiomalate (i.e., Au(I) oxidation state) are co-ordinated to two sulphur atoms with an Au–S bond length of 2.29 Å. This is consistent with the finding that the gold within particles obtained from rat kidney cells, in rats treated with long-term gold sodium thiomalate, is in the Au(I) oxidation state and is bound to two sulphur atoms with an Au–S bond length of 2.30 Å. The Au(I) oxidation state, therefore, appears to be the primary oxidation state in a biological milieu: reduction from Au(III) to Au(I) is probably caused by sulphydryl-containing reducing enzymes.

A common misconception is that D-penicillamine may be used as a chelating agent for gold, if a toxic reaction occurs during, or following, the administration of the anti-arthritic gold complexes. There is no theoretical or biochemical evidence that D-penicillamine chelates Au(I) *in vivo*. Indeed, Au(I) compounds normally have linear geometry in which the Au(I) atom is attached to two ligand atoms (X), such that the X–Au(I)–X angle is 180°. Less frequently, and for rather specific ligands only, Au(I) binds to three (X–Au(I)–X angle equal to 120°) or four (X–Au(I)–X angle equal to 109.5°)

ligand atoms. These three and four-coordinate complexes, with one exception, are only found with organic phosphine ligands and dipyridyl or O-phenanthroline. The only sulphur-containing compound to form a chelate and create a non-linear structure is a compound containing the tetrathiotungstate ion as a ligand. It is stabilized by an organophosphine. Thus, Au(I)–S bonds are at 180° to each other except in exceptional circumstances. Even when a ligand has two potential sulphur-bonding sites, the ligand binds to two different gold atoms rather than forming a chelate. One would expect D-penicillamine to bind Au(I) through the sulphydryl site only. Furthermore, Au(I) binds more readily to polarizable (soft) ligand groups such as sulphur or phosphine as opposed to weakly polarizable (hard) ligand groups, and the amine and carboxylate groups of D-penicillamine are 'hard'. Thus, there is no theoretical reason why D-penicillamine should chelate Au(I).

The anti-arthritic gold complexes and related structures

The gold complexes commonly used in the treatment of rheumatoid arthritis and in related research work are illustrated in figure 6.2.

Gold sodium thiomalate has been used in the treatment of rheumatoid arthritis for over 50 years. It is marketed in vials in which 50 mg/ml of the compound is suspended in sterile water for use as an intramuscular injection. The compound contains approximately 51% gold and 0.3 M of glycerol per mole of thiomalate. During the manufacturing process glycerol is used in the final purification step. The vials of compound marketed for human use also contain the following preservatives: phenylmercuric nitrate 0.002% (May and Baker preparation); chlorocresol 0.05% (Rhone–Poulenc preparation); benzyl alcohol 0.5% (Merck, Sharp and Dohme preparation). The currently assumed molecular weight of gold sodium thiomalate is 390.12. This value is based on the empirical formula of the compound, but clearly this structure is incompatible with the known chemical properties of Au(I) and the structure is probably a polymer or oligomer. Gold sodium thiomalate elutes from Sephadex G-100 as a polymeric structure and ultra-centrifuge and proton and carbon-13 nuclear-magnetic-resonance studies support this concept. Based on model building, a likely structural formula is a hexamer, although a pentameric structure has been suggested. Clearly the dearth of information on the structural formulation of gold sodium thiomalate, despite 50 years as a marketed drug, has contributed to the lack of knowledge of the biological interactions of this anti-arthritic complex and to determination of the definitive actions *in vivo* resulting in efficacy and toxicity. The simple formulation given as $Na_2[AuSCH(CO_2)CH_2CO_2]$ is inconsistent with the known chemistry of gold. The correct chemical name for gold sodium thiomalate, based on the structure given in the Martindale's Extra Pharmacopoeia is sodium (dithiomalato-S) aurate (I), but since the structure is almost certainly incorrect, the common term gold sodium thiomalate will be used throughout. No research group has

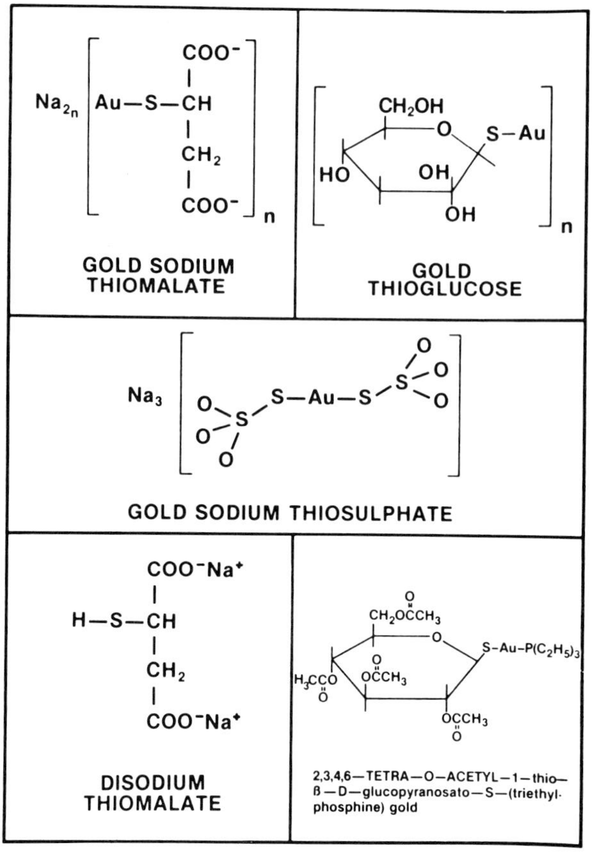

Figure 6.2. Gold complexes.

yet crystallized this compound so the determination of the crystal structure by X-ray diffraction has not been possible.

Gold thioglucose was manufactured in the USA by Merck Sharp and Dohme in the early 1930s. It is currently manufactured under the brand name Solganol by the Schering Corporation of New Jersey and is administered as an intramuscular injection. Although it is water-soluble, it is marketed as 50 mg of gold thioglucose in sterile sesame oil with 2% aluminium monostearate; 1 mg of propyl *p*-hydroxybenzoate is added as a preservative. The gold content is approximately 50.25% and the molecular weight based on the empirical formula is 392.18, but as with gold sodium thiomalate, the structural formulation is likely to be oligomeric.

Gold sodium thiosulphate is marketed as Sanochrysine in Europe by Nordisk and by Byk Gulden Lomberg Chemische, in vials of 100 mg of compound/ml, for use as an intravenous injection. The compound has a molecular weight of 490.21 and contains 40.19% gold. The anion contains two thiosulphate moieties which are bound to gold by their sulphur atoms. Gold sodium thiosulphate is one of the few Au(I) compounds whose structure is known and which has been studied crystallographically.

Gold sodium 3-thio-2-propanol-1-sulphonate is marketed in Europe as Allochrysine Lumière by Laboratoires de Therapeutique Moderne France. The manufacturer lists the gold content as being 30% but some analyses place the value as high as 52.9%. This variation may be dependent upon associated H_2O molecules or variations in the structural formulation of the gold compound during the manufacturing process (see discussion on gold sodium thiomalate). This compound is likely to be a small polymer. It was the original compound used by Forestier in 1928/29 and is still widely used in France, Switzerland and other parts of Europe.

Mercaptosuccinic acid is manufactured in the USA by Sigma Chemicals, St. Louis, Missouri and has a molecular weight of 150.15. The disodium thiomalate salt, in equimolar concentrations of thiomalate to gold sodium thiomalate, is prepared by the addition of 1 molar sodium hydroxide to the mercaptosuccinic acid solution (19 mg/ml) until a pH of 7.75 is achieved. The disodium salt is a monomeric species.

2,3,4,6-Tetra-O-acetyl-1-thio-β-D-glucopyranosato-S-(triethyl-phosphine) gold is manufactured as Auranofin™ by Smith, Kline and French, Philadelphia, USA. It is characterized by its gold–phosphine bond as well as its gold–thiol bond. Phosphines are usually bridging ligands and this accounts for the monomeric structure. It has been studied in a large number of clinical trials in the form of a 3 mg tablet. The compound is a white, odourless, crystalline solid which is insoluble in water. The powder is unstable and must be protected from light and heat. On a weight basis it contains approximately 29% gold and has a molecular weight of 678.5 and a melting point of 112–115°C.

Gold keratinate is manufactured in Germany as Aurodetoxin by Beecham-Wolfing. It is basically a gold–thiol structure attached to a polypeptide with the graphic representation of Au–S–R where R represents the polypeptide. The compound contains approximately 13% of Au(I). Gold distribution studies indicate that the gold from this compound binds predominantly to albumin (90%) with approximately 5% bound to macroglobulins. It is still widely used in Germany as an anti-arthritic agent.

Many other active Au(I)-thiol anti-arthritic agents have been developed in this century but the majority of research, both basic science and clinical, has been carried out on those described above.

Pharmacology of injectable gold compounds

The definitive mechanisms of action of the injectable gold compounds are unknown. *In vitro*, these gold–thiol compounds have been shown to inhibit prostaglandin synthesis and phagocytosis and to either kill or inhibit the growth of tubercle bacilli. The gold–thiol compounds are also known to inactivate the first components of complement (C_1) and to inhibit lysosomal enzymes such as acid phosphatase, beta-glucuronidase, elastase and cathepsin G. Gold sodium thiomalate, but no other gold compound, inhibits the action of the serine-esterase enzyme thrombin, both in vitro and *in vivo*. In view of the affinity of Au(I) for sulphur, the action of gold complexes against enzymes is most likely related to the large number of enzymes possessing an SH group in an easily accessible site. Gold sodium thiomalate appears to be particularly active against the serine esterase class (e.g., thrombin, which is phylogenetically related to elastase, trypsin and cathepsin G). It is probable that gold sodium thiomalate interacts with one, or all four, cysteine–cysteine bridges and thrombin molecule.

The administration of gold sodium thiomalate over a twelve-month period has been shown to be associated with a fall in all classes of immunoglobulin and rheumatoid factor titre. The gold complex has no effect on protein synthesis in general, since serum proteins remain constant and serum albumin levels rise. Gold sodium thiomalate has also been shown to inhibit the production of immunoglobulins in pokeweed-mitogen-stimulated immunoglobulin-secreting cells, but only when the gold complex was added to the culture on day one. This suggests that some aspect of macrophage function and/or T-helper-cell function is necessary for the production of this inhibitory effect. In terms of cytotoxicity, gold sodium thiomalate inhibits antibody-dependent, cell-mediated cytotoxicity when macrophages are used as effector cells; however, no such effect is seen when lymphocytes and polymorphs are used as effector cells.

Gold–sodium thiomalate has been shown to have a significant effect on the cell-mediated immune response *in vitro*. The addition of gold sodium thiomalate on day 1 of lymphocyte culture inhibits lymphocyte transformation to the mitogen phytohaemagglutinin and concanavalin A. It has been shown that this suppression of concanavalin-A lymphocyte transformation can be reversed by the addition of fresh peripheral blood monocytes, suggesting that the direct effect of the gold compound is on the monocyte, thus inhibiting the helper function of the macrophages to induce transformation. A similar effect is seen with mixed lymphocyte culture.

In summary, gold sodium thiomalate has an indirect effect on human B-cell function both *in vitro* and *in vivo*, probably owing to its inhibition of the human monocyte. This latter effect may be mediated through some inhibition of interleukin-1 production and/or function. It appears to have an effect on natural-killer-cell activity *in vitro*, but only for certain effector cells; it is difficult to correlate whether it has a specific effect on natural-killer cells *in vivo*. Gold sodium thiomalate inhibits both mitogen-stimulated lymphocyte responsiveness and mixed lymphocyte culture, provided it is added on day 1. Those people who respond to gold sodium thiomalate therapy regain normal mitogen and mixed-lymphocyte responsiveness, but whether the *in-vitro* response correlates with *in-vivo* effect is uncertain. It is of interest that injectable gold–thiol compounds inhibit certain viruses. If rheumatoid disease was ever identified as a chronic disease caused by Epstein–Barr virus or related viruses, one would have to consider the fact that the injectable gold–thiol compounds might work as an anti-viral agent.

Mechanism of action of Auranofin

The synthesis and development of Auranofin™, by Smith, Kline and French Laboratories, was an innovative approach to gold therapy.

However, the oral compound, Auranofin™, differs in many respects from the injectable gold–thiol compounds. The gold–thiol compounds, particularly gold sodium thiomalate are ubiquitous inhibitors of cellular enzymes, particularly serine-esterase enzymes. Auranofin™ does not inhibit these enzymes, but does prevent the release of lysosomal enzymes, such a beta-glucuronidase and lysozyme, from stimulated polymorphs.

Auranofin™ is a potent inhibitor of the antibody-dependent cellular cytotoxicity exhibited by polymorphs. In contrast, gold sodium thiomalate, gold thioglucose and the ligands of Auranofin™ have no significant effect on PMN-antibody-dependent cellular cytotoxicity. It is important to emphasize that the cellular viability, as assayed by trypan-blue exclusion, in these experiments was as great as 97% in the polymorph cultures, indicating that Auranofin™ did not induce cell death. Depending on the system used to study superoxide production, Auranofin™ is a much better inhibitor of superoxide production than gold sodium thiomalate. In certain systems (e.g., the immune phagocytosis system), gold sodium thiomalate was devoid of inhibitory activity at a concentration 40 times that of Auranofin™. In addition Auranofin™ is more potent than gold sodium thiomalate in the inhibition of cutaneous migration, chemotaxis and phagocytosis of peripheral blood monocytes. Like gold sodium thiomalate it inhibits lymphoblastogenesis *in vitro* by a direct inhibition of mononuclear-phagocyte function. This is achieved with concentrations of Auranofin™ which are 10–20-fold lower than those of the gold sodium thiomalate. In general, patients with active rheumatoid disease have a decreased capacity for either mitogen-stimulated lymphoblastogenesis or for lymphoblastogenesis produced by the mixed-lymphocyte reaction. Although patients initially treated with gold sodium thiomalate exhibit a suppression in mitogen-stimulated lymphoblastogenesis, those who eventually respond to the drug will show normal lymphocyte responsiveness *in vitro*. In contrast, within one week of patients receiving Auranofin™ lymphocyte responsiveness is markedly inhibited. This may reflect a major difference in the pharmacological properties of oral compounds versus the injectable gold–thiol compounds.

Pharmacokinetics of injectable gold compounds

Since the basic chemical structures of the commonly used injectable gold complexes are unknown, knowledge of their pharmacokinetic profiles is largely centred on the measurement of gold concentrations in plasma or urine. These compounds are not monomeric Au(I) salts, but are most likely small polymeric structures. Indeed gold sodium thiomalate is probably a mixture of complexes. For these reasons, interpretation or extrapolation of the drug effect based on the pharmacokinetics of gold alone should be observed with some degree of reservation.

The Au moiety of injectable-gold complexes is rapidly absorbed into the circulation following intramuscular injection. The standard dose of gold sodium thiomalate is 50 mg, once per week. Peak serum concentrations of 700–1000 μg/100 ml are achieved in 2–6 hours of injection. In the 6 days following these concentrations fall to around 300 μg/100 ml, demonstrating a 40% excretion of Au over the week. Approximately 75% of the Au is excreted via the kidney and the remainder in the faeces. During chronic dosing 33% of this excreted dose is derived from the most recent injection. If only one injection is given, lower percentages of gold are eliminated in the second and subsequent weeks, decreasing from 16% to 10%, by the sixth week. More than 95% of the administered gold is bound to albumin via the sulphur group on cysteine number 34. The remainder of the gold is bound to the macroglobulin layer (fraction I of electrophoresis). Radioactive-labelling studies of gold sodium thiomalate have shown that 50% of the ^{14}C label appears in the urine in 24 hours; it is unlikely that this represents intact thiomalate. Studies from the UK have revealed that even when purified gold sodium thiomalate has been produced, as much as 13% 'free thiomalate' may be detected in serum following an injection. As yet, no-one has determined what the active species is. Although there are studies to suggest that the amount of gold in the serum can be related to its effectiveness, the majority of authors do not find this to be the case. Indeed, the active species of the gold complex probably work at a cellular level.

The gold from injectable gold compounds is widely distributed throughout the reticulo-endothelial system particularly in the phagocytic cells of the liver, bone marrow, lymph nodes and spleen. Gold is also found in the synovium, but the site of deposition has given no indication as to the mechanism of action of the parent compound. Electron microscopic studies have demonstrated that the Au and S, located within the lysosomes of phagocytic cells, have a fibrillar-like appearance. Gold deposition in the skin is predominantly in the dermal area and there is a quantitative correlation between the amount of gold in the dermis and the total dose given. Electron-dense deposits of gold are also seen in the tubular cells of the kidney, another site rich in sulphydryl-containing enzymes, but the presence of gold associated with the glomerulus is extremely uncommon.

Gold levels have been detected in the milk of lactating mothers and in the serum and red blood cells of the nursing infant. The presence of the gold in the serum and red blood cells of the infant indicate that the chemical composition or binding of the Au, as presented to the infant, is in an orally absorbable form.

Pharmacokinetics of Auranofin

Phosphines are usually bridging ligands and this accounts for the monomeric structure of Auranofin. Like the gold–thiol compounds, Auranofin contains Au(I) only and binds to albumin via cysteine 34, the only sulphydryl group in albumin. When the sulphur atom is blocked, Auranofin will still bind to albumin, via nitrogen and will displace the chloride. Although the binding of gold sodium thiomalate to blood products is minimal *in vivo*, Walz and colleagues have shown that approximately 50% of the content of whole blood Au of Auranofin is the result of intracellular penetration in the red cells, the rest being associated with albumin. This membrane penetration of the red cells and lymphocytes is due to the lipophilic nature of the Auranofin molecule.

Following administration of ^{195}Au-labelled Auranofin, approximately 25% of the administered dose is detected in the plasma with peak concentrations of 6–9 μg/100 ml being reached in 1–2 hours. The majority of absorption takes place in the upper small bowel. The plasma half-life is in the order of 15–25 days with a total body elimination half-life of 55–80 days. This latter value is considerably less than that of gold sodium thiomalate. About 1% of ^{195}Au Auranofin is detectable by 180 days, whereas up to 30% of ^{195}Au from gold sodium thiomalate may be detected at this time. Single-dose kinetic studies, reveal that approximately 75–85% of ^{195}Au from Auranofin is detectable in the stool. This excretion continues slowly and, over a six-month period, the cumulative stool excretion of ^{195}Au may be as high as 88% of the original dose.

Clinical effects of injectable gold compounds

Uncontrolled studies, by Forestier and others, in the late 1920s suggested that gold was efficacious in the treatment of rheumatoid arthritis, but associated with adverse reactions. Lack of firm statistical evidence as to the usefulness of injectable gold compounds led the Empire Rheumatism Council in 1957 to plan a multi-centre trial. Ninety-nine patients in the treated group received 1000 mg of gold sodium thiomalate as 50 mg weekly injections over 20 weeks. One hundred control patients were given 0.01 mg of gold sodium thiomalate as 0.5 μg weekly over a 20-week period to form the placebo group. It was unequivocally demonstrated that in most patients given the 50 mg weekly gold sodium thiomalate, there was progressive improvement in a number of objective variables, including the number of joints clinically inflamed, grip strength and ESR. Although gold therapy was stopped after 20 weeks (1000 mg of compound), improvement persisted for up to 12 months in many patients and was generally maintained up to 18 months. However, by the thirtieth month (i.e., 24 months after gold therapy had been discontinued), little if any advantage was recorded.

In 1973, the Co-operating Clinic Committee of the American Rheumatism Association reported their double-blind trial of 68 patients with definite or classical rheumatoid arthritis. The initial phase of this study compared 36 patients, who received gold sodium thiomalate 50 mg weekly for six months, and a control group of 32 patients, who received sterile water vehicle over the same period. Twelve patients in the gold group dropped out because of adverse effects while another eight patients in the placebo group dropped out because of adverse effects and eight patients because of no benefit. The gold-treated group showed a slight, but definite, improvement in all parameters measured, although only the change in ESR was statistically significant. In the second phase of the study, designed to compare the results of maintenance therapy, patients received six 50 mg doses at two-week intervals for two years. Control patients received the sterile water vehicle in the same fashion. The gold group showed no increase in the number of involved joints, improved their grip strength and demonstrated a fall in ESR, but the control group deteriorated. The authors commented that the results of the Co-operating Clinics Committee Trial confirmed the findings of the Empire Rheumatism Council Trial and stated that the larger sample size of the latter allowed the differences recorded for grip strength and number of joints to reach statistical significance. However, it should be noted that, although both the patients in the Empire Rheumatism Council Trial and the Co-operating Clinics Committee Trial were comparable in almost all respects, there were marked differences in the category of duration of disease prior to therapy. The majority of patients in the Empire Rheumatism Council Trial had disease of less then three years duration and an upper limit of five years, whereas those in the Co-operating Clinics Committee Trial had no disease duration limit and almost one third of the patients had rheumatoid arthritis for longer than five years. Thus, if injectable gold works better when given early in the disease process, this would explain the greater demonstrable benefit seen in the Empire Rheumatism Council Trial.

The optimum dose for injectable gold has not been determined, although doses of 150 mg weekly have been shown to be no better, and significantly more toxic than 50 mg per week.

Recently there have been a number of trials suggesting that doses as low as 10 mg weekly may have a significant therapeutic effect in patients. There have been a number of attempts to correlate gold concentrations in serum with clinical efficacy, but the majority of these have failed to show any clear relationship and, although the question has not been answered clearly, it seems likely that the time and expense involved in monitoring these concentrations will not result in a major improvement in therapeutic efficacy. Clinical responses occurs in the first six months. Those who do not respond in this period are gold 'failures' and should be withdrawn. Complete remission however may not appear until 6–30 months.

Clinical effects of Auranofin

Auranofin has now had extensive short-term use in the treatment of rheumatoid arthritis. Dose–response studies have suggested that 9 mg daily causes unacceptable diarrhoea while 1 mg daily has no therapeutic effect. Recent studies have employed either 3 or 6 mg/day. A number of clinical trials have compared Auranofin with injectable gold salts and the results obtained have tended to suggest that gold sodium thiomalate and thioglucose act more rapidly and are probably clinically superior. However, Auranofin is associated with a spectrum of side-effects (diarrhoea) that less commonly lead to cessation of therapy, in contrast to those of the injectable gold compounds.

Side-effects of injectable gold compounds

The major limiting factor to the use of injectable compounds is toxicity. Approximately 30–50% of patients who receive an injectable gold compound will develop some form of toxicity. The most common side-effect is skin rash which occurs in approximately 30% of patients. This is usually represented by a dry itchy area, which is slightly erythematous and scaly in patches and the drug should be discontinued following its the development and not re-introduced until it has completely resolved. Once re-introduced, the drug should be administered in low doses of 10–25 mg weekly. Occasionally, severe skin rash develops which may lead to total exfoliation and intense pruritis.

Mouth ulcers occur in approximately 20% of patient and may, or may not, be painful. They resemble aphthous ulcers in appearance.

Approximately 20% of patients on injectable gold therapy will develop proteinuria at some stage. Proteinuria in excess of 1000 mg/24 hours necessitates the cessation of gold treatment and further investigation. The most common histological lesion is that of membranous glomerulonephritis, but tubular lesions can also be seen due to heavy metal damage. Once the proteinuria has reduced in quantity, gold therapy may be re-instituted at a lower dosage.

Although much less common than the above mentioned side-effects, myelotoxicity associated with gold therapy is the major cause of mortality. Thrombocytopaenia, defined as a decrease in platelet count below 150 000, occurs in approximately 10% of patients and there are two types. In the common variety the bone marrow contains abundant megakaryocytes and the mechanism of gold toxicity is thought to be due to an immune-mediated peripheral destruction of platelets. Surface-associated IgG is found on the platelet membrane and this type of thrombocytopaenia occurs with increased frequency in patients who are HLA-DR3-positive. It can occur at any time in the treatment course and has been seen in patients on maintenance therapy three to six years after starting the drug. The second type of thrombocytopaenia is due to bone-marrow depression. It occurs with larger doses of gold, may be preceded by a gradual reduction in platelet count and has a variable prognosis. Cessation of gold injections and, possibly, the administration of prednisolone, are often successful in restoring the platelet count to normal. Gold-induced neutropaenia and marrow aplasia with pancytopaenia are the most serious toxic effects of gold therapy, but are rare. Patients developing these exhibit a high mortality and there is little evidence that recovery is aided by corticosteroid therapy, dimercaprol or D-penicillamine. Bone-marrow suppression, or thrombocytopaenia, secondary to gold compounds is a contra-indication to further continuation of therapy. Most cases of serious blood dyscrasia can be avoided by the regular monitoring of blood counts and early cessation or reduction of gold dosage if the decreasing neutrophil or platelet count is noted on serial testing.

The immediate allergic or 'nitrotoid' reaction appears to be unique to the gold sodium thiomalate. It is manifest by flushing, sweating, headache, joint pains and hypotension and patients should be switched to either gold thioglucose or an oral gold compound if they find the reaction intolerable.

Other adverse reactions associated with gold therapy include colitis, pneumonitis, hepatitis and peripheral neuropathy. Gold colitis is rare, but important, because of its relatively high mortality. Gold-induced pneumonitis may present suddenly with onset of dyspnoea, crepitations and bilateral diffuse pulmonary shadowing on chest X-ray. Gold-induced hepatitis is also uncommon, manifests as intra-hepatic cholestasis, occurring after a small cumulative dose of gold, and is frequently associated with eosinophilia. Corneal chrysiasis is now well recognized by means of slit-lamp examination, but its presence does not require any alteration in treatment.

There is no apparent increase in the incidence of toxicity in elderly patients receiving gold compounds, although specific caution should be taken with regard to haematological toxicities since bone-marrow aplasia secondary to any drug is more commonly recorded in the elderly. Toxicity of injectable gold compounds and in particular renal side-effects are related to human-leucocyte-antigen tissue types. Patients with HLA-DR3 are more likely to develop toxic reactions to injectable gold sodium thiomalate and D-penicillamine. There is also a higher incidence of HLA-B8 in patients developing gold toxicity. However, patients possessing these antigens should not be denied therapy since the relative risk does not outweigh the potential clinical benefit.

Side-effects of Auranofin

The most common side-effect noted with Auranofin is diarrhoea, which tends to occur in up to 40% of patients. In most patients the frequency of bowel motions can be reduced by decreasing the dose of Auranofin. Skin rashes may also occur in up to 20% of patients, but only a small number have to discontinue therapy. Stomatitis occurs in 10–12% of patients and may also be associated with a skin rash. It is more likely to occur in the first month, but can be seen at any time. Although less common than with injectable gold therapy, proteinuria occurs in 2–3% of patients treated with Auranofin. In these cases, the drug should be withheld and assessments of renal function made. Rarely, thrombocytopaenia and bone-marrow suppression occur and in this situation, Auranofin should be withdrawn and not recommenced.

Gold treatment is usually monitored in the hope that early detection of side-effects and subsequent cessation or modification of gold dose will lead to recovery. Ideal management requires a complete blood picture and urinalysis for protein and blood to be performed before each gold injection or at monthly intervals during Auranofin therapy. Physicians who monitor gold treatment less frequently may miss the important downward trend in platelet or neutrophil count which often precedes bone-marrow aplasia. Thrombocytopaenia may occur suddenly and, therefore, it may not be detected by routine blood counts. However, if a consistent downward trend in platelet count is observed then gold therapy should be withheld until recovery occurs or an alternative cause for the thrombocytopaenia is discovered. Urine and blood tests should be entered into a log book which can be reviewed by the physician.

Drug interactions with gold

There are no significant interaction with Auranofin or the injectable gold compounds.

Summary of clinical guidelines

Gold therapy is indicated in the treatment of rheumatoid arthritis, polyarticular juvenile arthritis, psoriatic arthritis and palindromic rheumatism. There are very few contra-indications to the administration of gold compounds, but patients who have had a serious reaction to gold, particularly a haematological side-effect, should not be given the drugs. Gold injections are started in those patients who have failed to respond to an adequate trial of NSAIDs. An initial test dose of 10 mg is given on the first week, followed by 25 mg intramuscularly in the second week. Subsequently 50 mg is given intramuscularly for 20 weeks, followed by maintenance therapy every two to four weeks. Maintenance therapy is given for an indefinite period of time if serious side-effects do not occur. It should be discontinued if there is no response, toxicity, or the development of complete remission. Patients who have failed to respond to gold after six months of therapy are usually considered failures. Gold treatment can be expected to provide useful improvement in symptoms, at least in the short term, for between 60 and 80% of patients with rheumatoid arthritis. However, the time course of response is slow and benefit may not be seen for six months. The problem with gold therapy, as with other suppressive agents in rheumatoid arthritis, is that if patients are followed for a five-year period most patients will have ceased taking the drug either because of side-effects or relapse. Toxicity is the major cause of drop-out in the first 12 to 15 months of treatment with loss of efficacy producing a slow attrition rate after that. Long-term studies of Auranofin have not yet been completed, but with this lack of sustained long-term efficacy and the significant incidence of side-effects, gold therapy must continue to be viewed with respect.

D-Penicillamine

D-Penicillamine is a degradation product of penicillin and was isolated in the early 1940s. It is an amino acid containing a sulphydryl group and is chemically related to the naturally occurring amino acid L-cysteine. The proper chemical name for the substance is D-(−)-2-amino-3-mercapto-3-methylbutyric acid or 3,3-dimethylcysteine and it exists as D and L isomers, the former of which was found to be identical to naturally-derived penicillamine. Alkaline solutions of pure D-penicillamine are laevorotatory, hence D-penicillamine is correctly named D-(−)-penicillamine. The optical activity of the compound arises from the chiral α-carbon atom and in modern terminology D-penicillamine has the *S* configuration.

The D-penicillamine in use today has no antibiotic activity. It was first introduced, in 1956, by Walshe for the treatment of Wilson's disease and later used, in the early 1960s, in the treatment of cystinuria. Jaffe first used the drug in the treatment of rheumatoid arthritis in the early 1960s. The compound has been reported to be of value in a wide range of disorders such as rheumatoid arthritis, juvenile rheumatism, Wilson's disease, cystinuria, lead poisoning and radiation toxicity. Reports have also been published on its use in biliary cirrhosis, scleroderma, Duchenne muscular dystrophy, intra-ocular vitreous proliferation and haemolytic disease of the newborn. In addition it has been used as a ligand in the preparation of pharmaceuticals for liver and kidney imaging. Only D-penicillamine is used in medicine since the L isomer and the DL or racemate are toxic. Differences between the D and L penicillamine are shown in the ease with which they are incorporated into proteins and their activity with vitamin B_6. The structures of D-penicillamine and its major metabolites are shown in figure 6.3.

The principal mechanisms of action of D-penicillamine include thiazolidine formation, formation of disulphide links, chelation and the formation of metal complexes and superoxide dismutase-like activity. These chemical actions account for many of the beneficial and toxic reactions attributable to this compound.

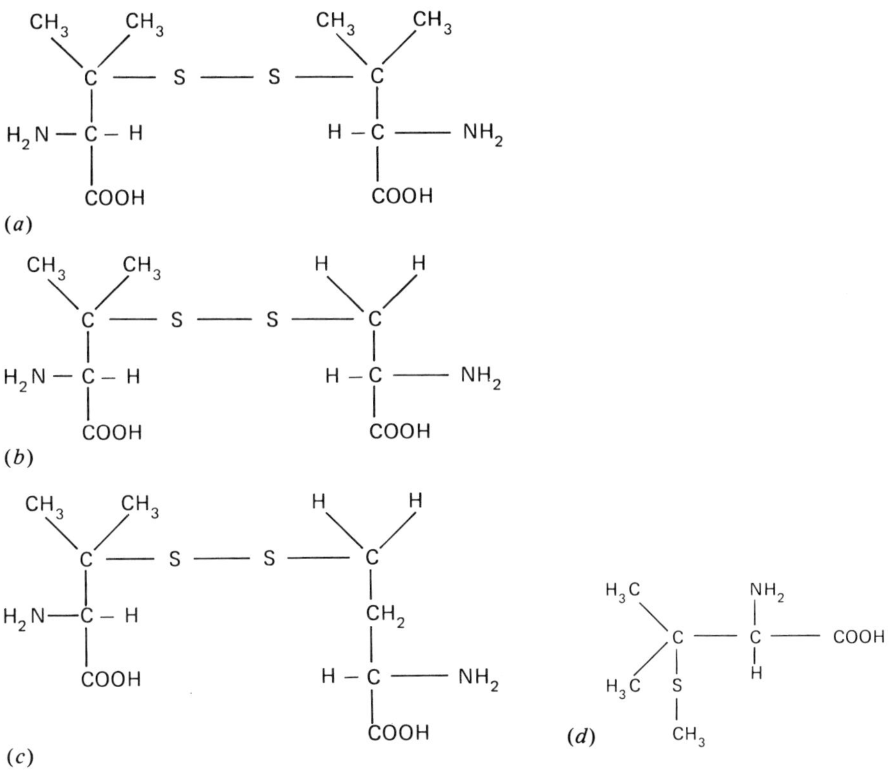

Figure 6.3. (*a*) Penicillamine disulphide, (*b*) penicillamine–cysteine disulphide, (*c*) penicillamine–homocysteine disulphide and (*d*) *S*-methyl-penicillamine.

Thiazolidine formation

D-Penicillamine is capable of crossing the placenta and its capacity to undergo the thiazolidine formation with maturing collagen makes it potentially teratogenic. Thiazolidine formation occurs when penicillamine condenses with carbonyl compounds (aldehydes and ketones) to give a substituted thiazolidine carboxylic acid (a closed five-membered ring) and water. During collagen synthesis penicillamine can inhibit or impair tropocollagen cross-linking between adjacent lysine and hydroxylysine residues by thiazolidine formation between the aldehyde group of lysine and the amino acid sulphydryl function of penicillamine. This interaction results in the formation of insoluble mature collagen. In theory, the chelating capacity of penicillamine could interfere with the function of lysine oxidase, a copper-dependent enzyme, and inhibit aldehyde formation, as in lathyrism.

Formation of disulphide links

D-Penicillamine is an essential form of treatment in cystinuria because of its capacity to undergo dimer formation, forming a disulphide link with cystine, which results in the formation of a water-soluble penicillamine–cysteine mixed disulphide. This compound is 50 times more soluble in urine than cystine and thus reduces the incidence and size of kidney-stone formation.

Chelation

Chelation (Greek: *Khele*, Latin: *Chele*, claw) is said to occur when two or more electron-pair donor sites from a polydentate ligand, for example penicillamine, attach to the same metal ion (for example copper, Cu) simultaneously and form a ring structure. Penicillamine is a versatile ligand since it has both 'hard' (weakly polarizable CO_2^- and $-NH_2$) and 'soft' (easily polarizable, S^-) binding sites available, depending on the pH of the reaction mixture. Metal binding to two or more of these sites results in the formation of a stable chelate ring. Penicillamine is the treatment of choice for hepato-lenticular degeneration (Wilson's disease) because of its ability to form stable complexes, through chelation, to copper and permit reduction in the excess non-protein bound copper in serum and tissues.

The chelating property of D-penicillamine has also been of value in the treatment of heavy-metal poisoning with mercury, cadmium and lead. Chelate complexes are also of use with $^{99}Tc^{m}$ for radio-imaging.

This knowledge that penicillamine is a metal chelator has led to two basic problems in the medical literature.

1. The assumption that penicillamine acts as a chelator for all metals including the gold (I) administered in gold–thiol complexes, for example gold sodium thiomalate.
2. The assumption that adverse effects occurring in patients receiving penicillamine might be related to penicillamine chelating previously-administered gold.

The first concept, that D-penicillamine chelates the Au (I) of gold sodium thiomalate is chemically incorrect (see page 92). Secondly, there is no clinical evidence that the previous administration of gold sodium thiomalate has an effect on the resulting efficacy or toxicity of D-penicillamine in patients with rheumatoid disease.

The ability of penicillamine to compete for Au(I) attached to protein is well established when excess penicillamine is present, but the D-penicillamine is probably bound only through a simple linear gold–sulphur bond. This type of competition appears not to be important at standard pharmacological doses. The evidence is against thiol-bound ligands, such as thiomalate, thioglucose, thiosulphate and D-penicillamine forming chelates with Au(I), and mobilization of bound gold *in vivo* by D-penicillamine through the mechanism of chelation is unlikely.

Superoxide dismutase-like activity

Superoxide dismutases are metallo-enzymes containing either copper, zinc, manganese or iron. Copper–penicillamine complexes have been shown to exhibit superoxide dismutase-like activity *in vitro*. The copper–zinc metallo-enzymes in human tissues are immunologically identical and are found in a large range of cell systems. During phagocytosis or the interaction of phagocytic cells with immune complexes and complement factors, active oxygen species (superoxide anion, hydrogen peroxide, hydroxyl radical and singlet oxygen) are produced. Newly-formed superoxide anion and hydrogen ion rapidly undergo dismutation to form hydrogen peroxide. It is this reaction which is catalysed by superoxide dismutases. All of these oxygen-derived species are potent oxidizing agents capable of inactivating sulphydryl enzymes breaking bonds in proteins, lipids and nucleic acids. Thus, it is theoretically possible that these oxygen-derived species are important mediators resulting in cellular damage during the inflammatory process. Penicillamine, especially as a copper complex, should theoretically protect against this aspect of inflammation by acting as a superoxide dismutase-like compound and accelerating the scavenging of superoxide anion. However, it is also reasonable to assume that the resultant hydrogen peroxide from this reaction is toxic to cellular tissue. This would explain why a copper–penicillamine complex might be responsible for T-lymphocyte inhibition to a greater extent than either copper sulphate or penicillamine alone.

Clearly the definitive mechanism of efficacy or toxicity of D-penicillamine in the treatment of rheumatoid disease remains to be elucidated, but many of its other chemical reactions can be demonstrated in the various disease states.

Chemistry and pharmacokinetics of D-penicillamine

D-Penicillamine is a white crystalline solid with a slight odour typical of sulphur-containing amino acids, and has a characteristic taste. It is relatively soluble in water at 10% w/w, slightly soluble in alcohol and almost insoluble in most common organic solvents. The compound is administered by the oral route and is rapidly absorbed from the upper gastro-intestinal tract. Absorption is reduced by the presence of food, antacids and iron in the diet. A 50% greater absorption has been identified in fasting, healthy volunteers. Absorption of the drug may be impaired by 33% with the concomitant use of an antacid, and up to 66% with the concomitant use of an iron preparation. Plasma concentrations of 15–20 μg/ml occur in 1–2 hours after ingestion. Approximately 80% of the administered D-penicillamine is bound to albumin, with smaller amounts bound to ceruloplasmin and other globulins. Small amounts occur as L-cysteine–D-penicillamine disulphide, free penicillamine, penicillamine disulphide and *S*-methyl-penicillamine. Plasma clearance follows a bi-phasic pattern with an early elimination phase of one to three hours followed by a much slower elimination with a half-life of approximately eight days. Approximately 33% of the drug is eliminated via the urine, 15% via faeces and as much as 33% degraded in the gut before absorption.

Clinical studies on D-penicillamine

In the late 1950s, it was reported that penicillamine, cysteine and several other thiol compounds caused macroglobulins to dissociate. Since rheumatoid factor is a macroglobulin, several investigators thought that penicillamine would dissociate rheumatoid factor. Jaffe confirmed that there was a decrease in the level of rheumatoid factor in the synovial fluid following intra-articular injection of D-sulphydryl compounds. He subsequently tested penicillamine in the treatment of rheumatoid disease. He showed that there was a gradual decrease in rheumatoid-factor titre with prolonged D-penicillamine administration, although this decrease was mainly confined to rheumatoid factor of the IgM class. In the early 1960s, Jaffe treated patients with rheumatoid disease for approximately 4–6 months and reported greater than 50% improvement in his patients, despite a high incidence of adverse effects. By the late 1960s Jaffe proposed that the use of lower doses and a more gradual introduction of D-penicillamine gave sufficient clinical efficacy but lower toxicity. The prescribing slogan of 'go low: go slow' was introduced and this regimen is now widely prescribed.

A number of trials have shown D-penicillamine to be better than a placebo. The optimal dosage regimen has not yet been determined although it seems that most patients require at least 500 mg/day for maximal effect.

Although it may be possible to reduce the dose of penicillamine in patients controlled on the drug, cessation of treatment is invariably associated with an exacerbation of disease activity.

Patients generally experience benefit from D-penicillamine after 8–12 weeks. Although over 60% of patients will derive some initial benefit from penicillamine treatment, this is not maintained over a five-year period, the majority of patients having disease exacerbation despite continuing therapy. The drug should not be denied to patients over the age of 60 as the elderly are as responsive as younger patients. The response to penicillamine is not influenced by initial starting dose, the rate of increase of dose, duration of disease or the absence or presence of seropositivity. There is no evidence that prior development of side-effects to gold sodium thiomalate will in any way influence either the efficacy or the toxicity experienced by patients receiving D-penicillamine. The indications for starting a patient on penicillamine are almost exactly the same as those indications for starting a patient on gold therapy. Any patient with rheumatoid arthritis who has not responded to a careful unhurried trial of NSAIDs should be offered the benefit of penicillamine. Most physicians give 125 mg/day for the first 4–8 weeks and increase this to 250 mg/day. With the more frequent availability of high-pressure liquid chromatography allowing better measurement of penicillamine levels, more accurate assessment of drug dosage will probably become available in the future. Some physicians increase the dosage to 750 mg/day, although the suggested evidence is that greater efficacy is not achieved at doses greater than 500 mg, and there is greater toxicity. During penicillamine therapy other medications such as NSAIDs and corticosteroids should be continued.

The majority of studies have indicated that penicillamine is as efficacious as injectable gold. The total incidence of adverse reactions on either treatment is no different, but the side-effects of penicillamine are perhaps less likely to cause withdrawal from treatment. Penicillamine has also been shown to be as effective as azathioprine in the treatment of rheumatoid disease though a higher incidence of drug withdrawal was noted in the azathioprine group, despite the fact there were more adverse effects on penicillamine. Penicillamine has also been shown to be as efficacious as chloroquine in a study which compared D-penicillamine, injectable gold and chloroquine. Penicillamine may be slightly more efficacious than Auranofin, although further studies are required to confirm this. Like injectable gold, it has been suggested that it may have the potential to induce remission and to favourably inhibit the radiological progression of erosions. Owing to the effect of penicillamine on collagen, reported above, it is now used in the management of patients with scleroderma, where it improves the skin elasticity. Theoretically, the earlier penicillamine is administered, the more likely it is to have a beneficial effect on the skin (see page 105).

D-Penicillamine has not been shown to be of any great value in the treatment of the sero-negative spondyloarthropathies although it has been used in the treatment of palindromic rheumatism with a reduction in the number of attacks.

There are no published double-blind, controlled trials to date on the use of D-penicillamine in juvenile arthritis. However, open studies have shown that D-penicillamine is as effective as injectable gold in children with juvenile rheumatism, showing a response rate of approximately 60–70%. This benefit was thought to be more specific for those children who were IgM sero-positive. Although to date there are few studies available as a guide to the use of D-penicillamine in juvenile arthritis, the overall frequency of efficacy from those children who have been treated is similar to that of adults, with an adverse reaction rate of approximately 20%. The usual recommended dose of D-penicillamine in children based on present studies is 15–30 mg/kg/day.

Side-effects

Only the D-isomer of penicillamine is available in therapeutic use and, although it is much less toxic than the L-isomer or the DL racemate, it has several adverse effects. The development of some side-effects, such as proteinuria, can be correlated with both dose duration and quantity of dose. However, the majority of side-effects can occur at any time. There is no clinical evidence that the adverse effects due to penicillamine in patients with rheumatoid disease are a reflection of the disease state, since side-effects such as skin rash, proteinuria and thrombocytopaenia, as well as the lupus-like reaction, occur in patients treated with penicillamine for Wilson's disease. In general, side-effects are most likely to occur in the first 18 months. As previously stated, previous gold therapy does not influence the development of adverse effects. There is, however, a possibile genetic basis for the increased susceptibility to adverse effects in those patients who have HLA antigens B8, DR2 and DR3.

SKIN RASH

The majority of skin rashes occur in the first 12 months and account for approximately 25–50% of all side-effects due to penicillamine. The majority of patients suffer a minor itchy, scaly rash of the hands, arms, trunk and legs. In many cases the rash is seen within the first three months of treatment. Elderly patients appear to have a greater chance of developing skin rash than younger patients. However, normal elderly patients do have a higher incidence of skin rash than the general population. The treatment of choice is to discontinue the penicillamine and treat the rash symptomatically, either with zinc ointment plus a suitable anti-pruritic agent, or, in more severe cases, topical corticosteroid. Erythema multiforme and a serum-sickness-type rash have also been described with penicillamine and may be seen in association with lymphadenopathy and mucosal involvement. In these cases, the drug should be discontinued immediately and, if necessary, oral corticosteroids prescribed. A skin rash of the bullous-type, resembling pemphigus, has been reported after six months of treatment and is usually referred to as 'the late rash'. Again the drug should be discontinued immediately and local anti-pruritics instituted. If the drug is withdrawn promptly the lesions usually resolve within one month, although persistent pemphigus has been reported. A maculopapular rash with a butterfly distribution may occur in the lupus-like syndrome and may be secondary to treatment with D-penicillamine. There are at least two reports of a characteristic rash which has disappeared when the drug has been withdrawn. Oral ulcers of the aphthous type occur with D-penicillamine, but are less common than with gold therapy. The presence of oral ulcers in a patient receiving penicillamine may precede the development of the pemphigus-like reaction. A penicillamine dermatopathy (skin thinning and friability over pressure points), elastosis perforans serpiginosa, excessive wrinkling of the skin and cutis laxa are rare side-effects and have been reported in patients with Wilson's disease or cystinuria. Other rare side-effects include lichen planus, epidermal inclusion cysts, morphea-like reaction, leukonychia, longitudinal nail ridge disruption and friability of finger nails.

TASTE ABNORMALITIES

Dysgeusia generally occurs in the first three to six months, with a variable incidence of 2 to 25% depending on the series of patients investigated. Most patients experience a sulphur or metallic-like taste. It was originally suggested that the abnormality may be due to a depletion of available zinc, but, studies of this trace metal have failed to confirm this. The taste abnormality will resolve and in general the patient does not have to discontinue the drug.

GASTRO-INTESTINAL TOXICITY

Gastro-intestinal toxicity has been reported as a side-effect of penicillamine and includes nausea, anorexia, abdominal pain and occasional diarrhoea. If all these symptoms are taken into account, the incidence is usually in the order of 8 to 35% but there is generally a higher incidence with increased dose. Gastro-intestinal disturbance usually occurs within the first six months, but may appear at any time. Symptoms are generally relieved by using either divided doses or a small reduction in dose. There is no evidence that D-penicillamine exacerbates peptic ulceration.

HEPATIC DYSFUNCTION

Liver-enzyme abnormalities occasionally occur in patients on penicillamine, but resolve on discontinuation of the drug. No deaths or cases of irreversible liver failure have been reported. Cholestatic hepatitis and frank jaundice have also been reported with D-penicillamine therapy.

HAEMATOLOGICAL EFFECTS

The most common haematological side-effect is thrombocytopaenia due to a the suppression of platelet production in the bone marrow. To date there are no recorded instance of platelet surface-associated, IgG-type thrombocytopaenia. The risk of thrombocytopaenia increases with higher doses and at the time a dose is increased. Since the fall in platelet count is gradual, a downward drift in platelet count should be taken as a warning sign of impending bone-marrow suppession. Thrombocytopaenia can occur at any time, but is generally seen in the first six months. If the platelet count drops below 150 000, the drug should be withheld until two consecutive platelet counts indicate that the absolute platelet count is stable and that there are no other associated haematological abnormalities of the white or red cells. Patients who have severe bone-marrow suppression and thrombocytopaenia should not be given D-penicillamine again.

A decrease in leucocyte count is much less common. The exact mechanism is not defined, but it is evident that it is due to a decrease in production from the bone marrow. It is uncommon for neutropaenia to occur precipitously, and like thrombocytopaenia, it is usually preceded by a gradual fall in white-cell count. In 1979 eight of ten deaths from D-penicillamine were related to blood dyscrasias — one from thrombocytopaenia, two from marrow aplasia and five from white-cell suppression. In seven of these cases, demonstrable warning falls in platelet and neutrophil counts were present. Bone-marrow recovery in the survivors took up to one year. It is therefore our recommendation that D-penicillamine be withheld if the leucocyte count falls below 4000 mm^3 or if there is a fall in neutrophil count below 2000 mm^3 and/or a rise in the absolute monocyte count above 500 mm^3. Patients who have developed significant neutropaenia secondary to D-penicillamine should not be re-challenged with the drug.

Rarely haemolytic anaemia, sideroblastic anaemia, transient eosinophilia, thrombocytosis and polycythaemia have been reported in association with D-penicillamine.

Immunoglobulin decreases have been reported in patients with Wilson's disease and there are also reports of IgA deficiency. However, there is at least one report of the successful and safe use of penicillamine in patients with sero-negative rheumatoid arthritis with concomitant IgA deficiency. Immune complexes have been shown to decrease during penicillamine therapy, as has the α-1-anti-trypsin–IgA complex. IgM rheumatoid factor decreases during penicillamine therapy and, to a lesser extent, so does IgG rheumatoid factor.

Renal toxicity

Proteinuria secondary to penicillamine has been reported in patients with rheumatoid disease, cystinuria and Wilson's disease. It occurs in approximately 30% of all patients who receive the drug and is most common between the sixth and fifteenth month. The risk of proteinuria is higher with higher doses. Patients who carry HLA-B8 and -DR3 are apparently at greater risk of developing proteinuria secondary to penicillamine, but there is no evidence that this is more common in elderly patients. If the proteinuria is less than 500 mg/day, the drug may be continued, but if it is in the range of 500 to 3000 mg/day, the drug should be withheld until full renal function is assessed. If proteinuria is greater than 3000 mg/day the drug should be discontinued. Approximately 25% of patients who develop proteinuria greater than 3000 mg/day will have a frank nephrotic syndrome. In these patients the drug should be withheld although it should be noted that while permanent renal insufficiency is rare, the patient may continue to spill protein for one or two years, before the condition resolves. The histological lesion in the kidney is a membranous glomerulonephritis. The electron microscopy of renal biopsy tissue usually reveals subepithelial electron-dense deposits and the fusion of epithelial foot process. The immunofluorescent microscopy demonstrates granular capillary wall deposits of IgG and C3. These histological abnormalities may persist for up to one year after the withdrawal of the penicillamine. Less commonly, haematuria is seen, and the drug should be stopped immediately and the cause investigated with full assessment of renal function and cystoscopy.

Autoimmune syndromes

Although the majority of side-effects resemble those of the gold–thiol drugs, a feature of penicillamine therapy is the large number of autoimmune reactions. Patients have been recorded with serum sickness-like illness, lupus-like syndrome, Goodpasture's-like pulmonary–renal syndrome, pemphigus, myasthenia gravis, polymyositis, dermatomyositis and haemolytic anaemia. Autoimmune thyroiditis with high-titre thyroid antibodies have also been reported.

The lupus-like syndrome may occur at any time during the course of penicillamine treatment and is not dose-dependent. It was first reported in a patient with Wilson's disease, suggesting that patients do not require a pre-disposition to an autoimmune disorder in order to develop such a complication. The clinical presentation varies from the development of a positive anti-nuclear factor with lymphadenopathy, to a full-blown severe illness with widespread joint pain, synovitis, skin rash, malaise, weight loss nephritis, pleurisy and neurological disturbances. The anti-DNA binding antibody and lupus band test may be positive in these patients. As many as 25% of patients will develop a positive anti-nuclear factor when given penicillamine, although the clinical features of a lupus-like reaction probably occur in less than 2% of all patients. The disease process resolves within two to four months of drug withdrawal. There is at least one report which states that patients with HLA-A11 and -B15 are at greater risk of developing this side effect.

More than 60 cases of D-penicillamine-induced myasthenia-like syndrome have been reported in patients with rheumatoid disease, scleroderma and Wilson's disease. Although myasthenia gravis itself can occur in patients with rheumatoid disease, the syndrome which develops secondary to penicillamine differs in several aspects. First, the condition usually resolves on withdrawal of the drug, and second, the anti-acetylcholine-receptor antibody, which develops in patients with myasthenia gravis secondary to penicillamine, has been shown to be more specific and to have a higher affinity than that occurring in idiopathic disease. The titre of anti-acetylcholine-receptor antibodies decrease in the majority of patients after withdrawal of penicillamine and can be used as an indication of resolution. The usual clinical manifestations, include weakness of the ocular, bulbar, trunk, limb and respiratory muscles. Treatment involves withdrawal of the penicillamine and the institution of anti-cholinesterases, although in some cases, steroids, thymic irradiation, thymectomy and even plasmapheresis have been used. Symptoms may persist for up to a year after discontinuation of therapy, but the majority of cases will resolve within the first one or two months. A third factor which distinguishes the myasthenia gravis-like syndrome secondary to penicillamine from idiopathic forms is the higher prevalence of HLA-B35 and-DR 1 in the former compared to high incidence of HLA-B8-DR3 in patients with idiopathic myasthenia gravis.

A Goodpasture's-like syndrome characterized by haemoptysis and haematuria with progressive renal insufficiency has been observed in patients receiving D-penicillamine for Wilson's disease and rheumatoid arthritis. Antiglomerular basement-membrane antibody and the linear pattern of immunofluorescence on renal biopsy is not seen in these patients, hence, the condition is not a true Goodpasture's syndrome. The syndrome seems to be caused by immune-complex-mediated tissue injury, rather than tissue-directed antibody damage. In all other respects the Goodpasture's-like syndrome resembles the idiopathic condition with pulmonary infiltrates, haemoptysis, fever, haematuria and red cell casts and progressive renal insufficiency. No deaths have been reported. Early intervention with discontinuation of therapy generally results in resolution of the disease state within six to eight weeks.

Other lung problems, such as diffuse alveolitis presenting as bilateral pulmonary infiltrates and the development of an obliterative bronchiolitis, have been reported.

There are several case reports of dermatomyositis and polymyositis in association with penicillamine. However, these conditions are more likely to be a polymyopathy characterized by weakness and lymphocytic infiltration of muscle tissue. There are no case reports of frank muscle necrosis seen secondary to penicillamine, and the histopatholgy of skin biopsy speciments in penicillamine-induced dermatomyositis are not similar to those of the idiopathic condition.

MISCELLANEOUS SIDE-EFFECTS

There are now several reports in the literature of mammary gigantism associated with D-penicillamine. Patients usually experience a painful breast enlargement which resolves gradually after drug withdrawal. Reversible gynaecomastia has also been recorded in male patients. Other side-effects include photophobia, blurred vision, optic neuritis, neuromyotonia, hot flushes and peripheral neuropathy.

Toxicity monitoring

Patients who are started on penicillamine therapy should be seen regularly for careful drug monitoring in order to record benefit and/or toxicity related to the drug. It is generally recommended that the patients have a complete blood count, ESR and urinalysis every week for the first four weeks, every two weeks for the next two months and thereafter monthly. If the patient develops any of the side-effects mentioned above, the drug should be withheld until confirmation of the association of the side-effect with it is made. Patients should be initially started on 125 mg/day for the first 4–8 weeks and the dose gradually increased to 500 mg/day. There is no good evidence to date that doses greater than 500 mg will afford greater benefit, although it is well recognized that doses higher than 500 mg/day are associated with a more frequent incidence of toxicity.

Although D-penicillamine is a hydrolysate of penicillin, cross-sensitivity is extremely rare. Only in those patients who have had previous life-threatening anaphylactoid reactions to penicillin would one consider skin testing before the administration.

D-Penicillamine tablets should be administered with water and should be taken on an empty stomach, at a time as far removed from meals as possible. No other drugs should be taken concomitantly, especially iron supplements. Patients with Wilson's disease who become pregnant require D-penicillamine therapy to continue, since discontinuation results in a higher incidence of foetal wastage, but those patients with cystinuria and rheumatoid arthritis who become pregnant should have the drug withdrawn, if possible, since there are case reports of children being born with hypotonia and hyporeflexia.

Summary of clinical guidelines

D-Penicillamine is indicated in the early management of inflammatory rheumatoid disease which has not responded to maximum treatment with NSAIDs. The drug should be started at a low dosage (125 mg) and slowly increased over 8–12 weeks to a maximum of 500 mg/day. The drug should be given to co-operative and reliable patients only. The patient should be followed on a monthly basis in order to record drug effectiveness and a toxicity-monitoring chart used to document and intercept any adverse effects. D-Penicillamine has been shown to be as efficacious as injectable gold, azathioprine and the anti-malarials and, therefore, they can be used interchangeably. This drug is just as effective in the elderly as it is in the young, and, in the studies which have been done, it appears that only skin rash and taste abnormality are increased in the elderly.

Other thiols

Since the demonstration of efficacy of D-penicillamine in rheumatoid arthritis, a number of other thiol compounds such as pyrithioxine and 5-thiopyridoxine (figure 6.4) and captopril (figure 6.5) have been used.

Pyrithioxine and 5-thiopyridoxine have both been shown to be efficacious in the treatment of rheumatoid arthritis. These compounds seem to have a different mechanism of action from D-penicillamine in that they have little effect on copper excretion or vitamin B_6 metabolism. Recent open studies of these two compounds, in patients with rheumatoid arthritis, have demonstrated similar clinical effects to those of D-penicillamine with a slow onset of action and a similar spectrum of side-effects.

The specific angiotensin-converting-enzyme inhibitor captopril has also been shown to suppress rheumatoid arthritis in a small number of patients. Captopril diminishes lymphocyte responses to a variety of mitogens and this in part may explain its anti-arthritic effect. Side-effects of captopril are also

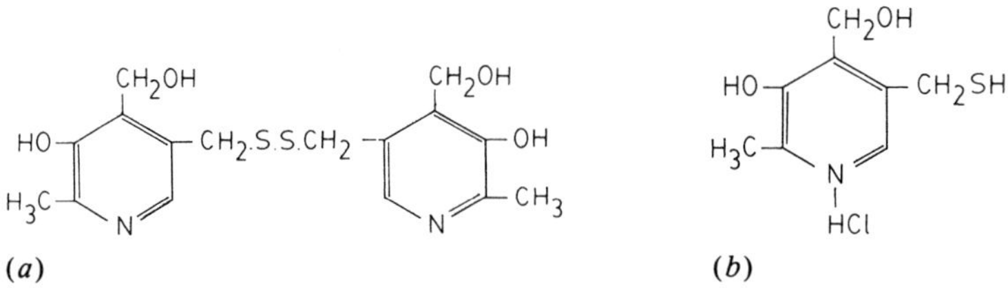

Figure 6.4. (*a*) Pyrithioxine and (*b*) 5-thiopyridoxine.

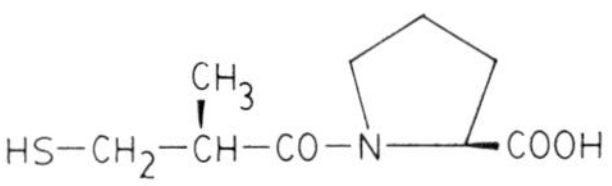

Figure 6.5. Captopril.

similar to D-penicillamine with skin rashes, transient taste disturbances, nephrotic syndrome and haematological side-effects being most common.

The demonstration of efficacy of these compounds in patients with rheumatoid arthritis underlines the importance of studying thiol compounds in an effort to find others with D-penicillamine-like activity.

Sulphasalazine

Sulphasalazine is a conjugate of 5-aminosalicylic acid, a salicylate analogue, and sulphapyridine, a sulphonamide, linked by an azo bond (figure 6.6). Approximately 23 to 33% of the drug is absorbed from the upper gastro-intestinal tract, with peak serum concentrations being reached after three to four hours, and steady-state serum levels after 24 hours. Approximately 10% of sulphasalazine is absorbed and excreted either unchanged in the urine or in the bile (enterohepatic circulation). The mean elimination half-life, after a single dose, is about six hours, and, after repeated doses, about eight hours.

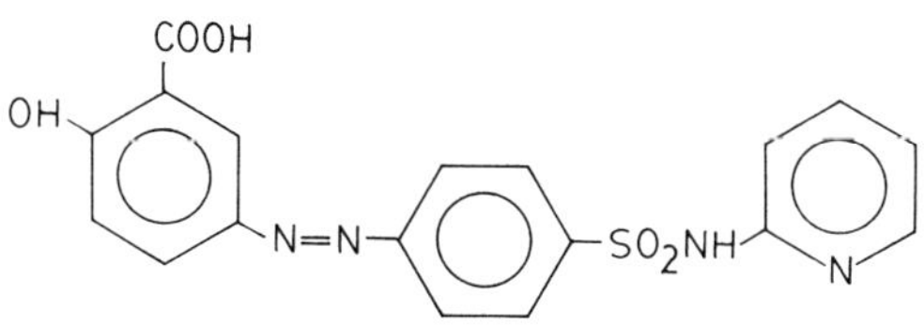

Figure 6.6. Sulphasalazine.

Mode of action

The mode of action of sulphasalazine is not known. Since only 10% of sulphasalazine is absorbed and serum concentrations bear no relationship to clinical effect in ulcerative colitis, it seems unlikely that sulphasalazine itself is the active moiety. There are conflicting reports on the relationship of serum concentrations of sulphapyridine to clinical response in ulcerative colitis, and current evidence favours 5-aminosalicylate as the active substance in this disease. Whether the action of 5-aminosalicylate causes an alteration in bowel flora or a local anti-inflammatory action is not known.

Clinical studies, both controlled and uncontrolled, have shown that sulphasalazine has a second-line effect in rheumatoid arthritis, and that the toxicity profile is less than other second-line drugs. However, the way in which sulphasalazine exerts its effect in rheumatoid arthritis remains a mystery but it may be related to the thiol group in the sulphapyridine ligand. The small amount of sulphasalazine absorbed from the colon is insufficient to inhibit prostaglandin synthesis in the joints. There is evidence, however, that the drug modulates various aspects of immune responses, but its relevance is uncertain.

Metabolism

In humans, the initial step in sulphasalazine metabolism occurs in the colon where the intestinal bacteria possess an intracellular azo-reductase, inhibited by oxygen, that reduces the azo bond of the molecule, releasing 5-aminosalicylate and sulphapyridine.

After azo-bond reduction most of the sulphapyridine is absorbed from the colon and partially acetylated and/or hydroxylated in the liver and/or conjugated with glucuronic acid. The remaining free sulphapyridine and its acetyl and glucuronide derivatives are then excreted in the urine.

After oral administration of sulphasalazine, sulphapyridine can be detected in the blood some three to five hours later, a time consistent with the transit time to the colon. Like hydralazine and isoniazid, sulphapyridine is subject to polymorphic acetylation, patients who are slow acetylators having higher free serum-drug concentrations than fast acetylators. Non-acetylated sulphapyridine is protein bound, reaching a maximum serum concentration after 12 hours, and taking some three days to clear from the serum after the drug is discontinued.

Most of the 5-aminosalicylic acid is excreted in the faeces, only a small amount being absorbed from the colon and excreted in the urine, mostly as the acetylated derivative. There is some evidence that 5-aminosalicylic acid may be subject to intestinal wall, as well as systemic, acetylation. It is of interest that when sulphapyridine and 5-aminosalicylic acid are administered separately by mouth, both are absorbed in the small intestine and excreted in the urine.

Sulphasalazine and its metabolites cross the placenta and can readily be detected in foetal tissue. There is no evidence, however, that this is harmful to the foetus. Likewise, sulphasalazine and sulphapyridine pass readily into milk, but to date no reports of kernicterus or other side-effects have been reported in breast-fed infants.

Drug interactions

Drug interactions occur in the gut or following absorption. Cholestyramine binds to sulphasalazine and its azo reduction products in the gut. Sulphasalazine chelates iron, and oral iron reduces sulphasalazine absorption. Calcium gluconate slows the absorption of sulphasalazine, but has no effect on the quantity absorbed. Broad-spectrum antibiotics reduce the bacterial degradation of sulphasalazine. Impairment of folic-acid absorption by sulphasalazine has been observed in patients with inflammatory bowel disease and in normal volunteers. Phenobarbitone decreases acetylsulphapyridine and serum sulphasalazine levels, but leads to an increase in hydroxy-sulphapyridine. There is no information on whether sulphapyridine, which is strongly protein bound, displaces other highly bound drugs such as oral anti-coagulants and anti-diabetic agents.

Side-effects

There is considerable variation in the incidence of side-effects from sulphasalazine, estimates ranging from 15 to 70%. The incidence is related to the dose of sulphasalazine, serum sulphapyridine levels, and acetylator status. The commonest side-effects are anorexia, nausea, vomiting and headache. Heartburn, epigastric pain, and diarrhoea may also occur, as may tinnitus and vertigo.

Rashes are usually mild but occasionally serious rashes may occur, such as exfoliative dermatitis, Stevens–Johnson syndrome and epidermal necrolysis (Lyell's syndrome). Cyanosis, which is not related to dimished oxygen-carrying capacity of haemoglobin or to methaemoglobinaemia, may occur also.

A variety of hepatic complications have been reported, including a reaction resembling acute viral hepatitis with very high concentrations of serum transaminase, cholestasis with marked hyperbilirubinaemia and elevated alkaline phosphatase, granulomatous hepatitis, and a mixed picture with mild to moderate elevations of bilirubin, alkaline phosphatase and transaminase levels. Hepatitis has been accompanied in most patients by fever and skin rashes. Corticosteroid therapy may be required, but total resolution of the hepatitis usually occurs on withdrawal of the drug. Reversible pancreatitis has been reported also.

Respiratory complications have included a clinical and radiological picture resembling eosinophilic pneumonia, with cough, fever, dyspnoea and weight loss beginning some two to five months after starting sulphasalazine. Eosinophilia and peripheral pulmonary infiltrates are invariably present. Complete resolution of all the clinical and laboratory abnormalities occur on discontinuing therapy. A fatal dose of sub-acute fibrosing alveolitis has been reported with treatment with sulphasalazine. Laryngotracheitis with bronchospasm has been noted and tachycardia may occur soon after dose administration.

The commonest haematological complication is haemolytic anaemia, which is usually mild and well compensated, with reticulocytosis as the sole laboratory abnormality. Haemolytic anaemia has also been reported associated with glucose-6-phosphate dehydrogenase deficiency, Heinz bodies, methaemoglobinaemia, and sulphaemoglobinaemia. Megaloblastic anaemia secondary to folic-acid deficiency has been reported, as has red cell aplasia. Neutropaenia and thrombocytopaenia are rare, but potentially serious complications.

Allergic reactions with fever, skin rashes, facial oedema, arthralgia and nephrotic syndrome occasionally occur. A drug-induced lupus syndrome has been described, as has Raynaud's phenomenon. Reversible peripheral neuropathy has been reported as has oligospermia, which rapidly recovers on drug withdrawal.

There is good evidence that certain of the side-effects are dose related (e.g., nausea, vomiting and headache). These are almost certainly due to sulphapyridine, and are more common in slow acetylators. Many of the other side-effects such as fever and skin rashes appear to be 'allergic' in nature, and desensitization regimens have proved useful in re-introducing drug treatment.

Levamisole

Levamisole (figure 6.7), was originally introduced as an antihelminthic, but has been shown to be effective in rheumatoid arthritis in a number of controlled trials.

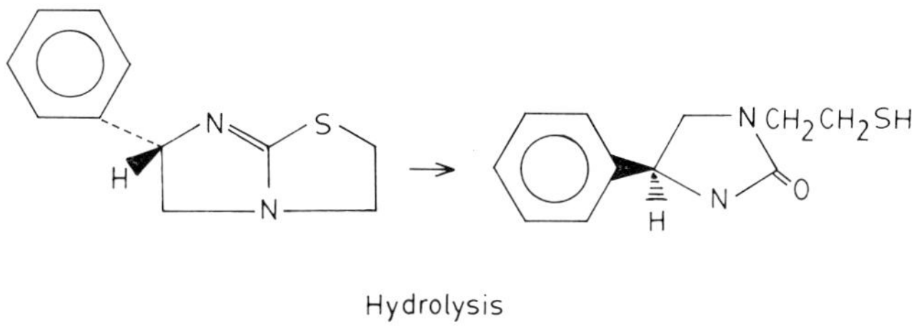

Figure 6.7. Levamisole hydrolysis to OMPI.

Mechanism of action

The mode of action of levamisole is complex and somewhat unclear. At very high doses the drug has anti-inflammatory properties, but these seem to be mediated by adrenal corticosteroids. At therapeutic doses levamisole has no anti-inflammatory action.

The effects of levamisole on the immune system have not been entirely defined. There is evidence that it has a dual spectrum of activity: it stimulates precursor T lymphocytes to differentiate into mature T cells and restores the normally depressed-effector functions of peripheral T lymphocytes and phagocytes. Levamisole restores delayed skin reactions in elderly persons and in patients with immunodeficiency. B cells are not stimulated by levamisole directly and the drug has no direct effect on antibody production.

The effects of levamisole and those of thymic hormones are similar and it has been suggested that levamisole might interact with thymopoietin receptor sites on lymphocytes, PMNs and macrophages, especially as there is a structural similarity between levamisole and the active site of the thymopoietin pentapeptide. However, levamisole has a sulphur-containing ring, and can be easily hydrolysed into OMPI (*dl*-2-oxo-3-(2-mercaptoethyl)-5-phenyl-imidazolidine), which contains a free sulphydryl group. Levamisole may enhance leucocyte functions through OMPI, by scavenging deleterious oxygen radicals and enhancing microtubule integrity.

Pharmacokinetics

The drug is rapidly absorbed from the gastro-intestinal tract, peak plasma concentration occurring within one or two hours. It is extensively metabolized in the liver, the plasma elimination half-life being approximately four hours, and completely eliminated from the body within two days.

Clinical effects

Levamisole is effective in rheumatoid arthritis. However, as with other second-line agents, the clinical benefits are not apparent for six weeks to three months, with a maximum effect being seen between six and 12 months. Clinical improvement is accompanied not only by a rise in haemoglobin and haematocrit concentrations and a fall in ESR, but also by a fall in rheumatoid-factor titre and a reduction in acute-phase reactants. A higher incidence of cold lymphocytotoxic antibodies has been reported during treatment, but there is no evidence that other auto-antibodies develop. Delayed hypersensitivity reactions of the skin are restored, reduced E-rosette numbers are increased and excessive EAC-rosette or null-cell numbers are reduced to normal. Neutrophil chemotaxis and the inhibition of the migration of leucocytes are enhanced, while the phagocytic activity of PMNs is increased. The response of lymphocytes to phytohaemagglutinin is inconsistent. Restoration of immunological abnormalities occurs soon after treatment with levamisole is begun, but does not correlate with clinical benefit.

The clinical response to levamisole appears unrelated to age, sex, duration of disease, use of NSAIDs and disease severity at the start of treatment. Initially, levamisole was prescribed at doses of 150 mg/day, but 150 mg three times weekly was found to be just as effective, and now 150 mg/week is recommended. The dose does not require adjustment for body weight, at least in adults. No therapeutic trials have been carried out in other rheumatic diseases.

Side-effects

Side-effects account for most of the patients withdrawing from treatment. Rash is the most frequent side-effect and usually clears up with discontinuation of therapy. Rarely, a vasculitic purpura may develop. An influenza-like illness and stomatitis may occur also. Intercurrent virus infections, such as chicken pox, may be extremely severe in patients receiving treatment with levamisole. However, the most serious side-effect, is agranulocytosis, which appears to be more common in HLA-B27 individuals. Agranulocytosis can occur with great rapidity, shortly after the start of treatment. Unlike gold and D-penicillamine, levamisole does not cause nephropathy. There are no known drug interactions either.

Further reading

Proceedings of a symposium — a reassessment of plaquenil in the treatment of rheumatoid arthritis, 1983 *American Journal of Medicine*, July 18, **75**(1A).

Day, R. O., Sambrook, P., Champion, G. D. and Graham, G. G., 1982, Antimalarials in rheumatic diseases. *Australian and New Zealand Journal of Medicine*, **12**, 645–649.

Mackenzie, A. H., 1983, Anti-malarial drugs for rheumatoid arthritis. *American Journal of Medicine*, Dec. 30, **75**(6A), 48–58.

Mackenzie, A. H. and Scherbel, A. L., 1980, Chloroquine and hydroxychloroquine in rheumatological therapy. *Clinics in Rheumatic Diseases*, **6**, 545–566.

Chaffman, M., Brogden, R. N., Heel, R. C., Speight, T. M. and Avery, G. S., 1984, Auranofin. *Drugs*, **27**, 378–424.

Champion, G. D., 1984, Gold compounds in rheumatic diseases—1. *Medical Journal of Australia*, **140**, 73–77.

Gibbons, B., 1979, Complications of crysotherapy. *Archives of Internal Medicine*, **139**, 343–346.

Proceedings of Conference: Therapeutic Innovation in Rheumatoid Arthritis, 1982, edited by P. Davis, and M. Harth, *Journal of Rheumatology*, (*Supplement 8*).

Smith M. D. and Brooks, P. M., 1984, Gold compounds in rheumatic disease — 2, *Medical Journal of Australia*, **140** 77–81.

References

Brooks, P., M., Miners, J. O., Smith, K. Smith, M. D., Fearnley, I. D. and Birkett, D. J., 1984, Dose plasma concentration and response relationships of D-penicillamine in patients with rheumatoid arthritis. *Journal of Rheumatology*, **11**, 772–775.

Bunch, T. W., O'Duffy, J. D., Tompkins, R. B. and O'Fallon, W. M., 1984, Controlled trial of hydroxychloroquine and D-penicillamine singly and in combination in the treatment of rheumatoid arthritis. *Arthritis and Rheumatism*, **27**, 267–276.

Huskisson, E. C., Jaffe, I. A., Scott, J. and Dieppe, P. A., 1980, 5-Thiopyridoxine in rheumatoid arthritis: clinical and experimental studies. *Arthritis and Rheumatism*, **23**, 106–110.

Jaffe, I. A., 1983, Thiol compounds with penicillamine-like activity and possible mode of action in rheumatoid arthritis. *Antirheumatic Drugs*, edited by E. C. Huskisson (Praeger) pp. 555–568.

Kean, W. F., Dwosh, I. L. Anastassiades, T. P., Ford, P. M. and Kelly, H. G., 1980, The toxicity pattern of D-penicillamine therapy. *Arthritis and Rheumatism*, **23**, 108–164.

Kean, W. F., Bellamy, N. and Brooks, P. M., 1983, Gold therapy in the elderly rheumatoid patient. *Arthritis and Rheumatism*, **26**, 705–711.

Kean, W. F., Kassam, Y. B., Lock, C. J. L., Buchanan, W. W., Rischke, J. and Nablo, L., 1984, Antithrombin activity of gold sodium thiomalate. *Clinical Pharmacology and Therapeutics*, **35**, 627–632.

Kean, W. F., Bellamy, P., Lock, C. J. C. and Adachi, J., 1984, Bio-inorganic effects of D-penicillamine in children and in the elderly. *Clinical Investigative Medicine*, **7**, 77–83.

Lyle, W. H., 1979, Penicillamine. *Clinics in the Rheumatic Diseases*, **5**, 569–601.

Martin, M. F. R., McKenna, F., Bird, H. A., *et al.*, 1984, Captopril: A new treatment for rheumatoid arthritis. *Lancet*, **1**, 1325–1327.

Neumann, V. C., Grindulis, K. A., Hubball, McConkey, B. and Wright, V., 1983, Comparison between penicillamine and sulphasalazine in rheumatoid arthritis: Leeds–Birmingham Trial. *British Medical Journal*, **287**, 1099–1102.

Paulus, H. E., Williams, H. J., Ward, J. R. *et al.*, 1984, Azathioprine versus D-penicillamine in rheumatoid arthritis patients who have been treated unsuccessfully with gold. *Arthritis and Rheumatism*, **27**, 721–727.

Pullar, T. and Capell, H. A., 1984, Sulphasalazine. A new anti-rheumatic drug. *British Journal of Rheumatology*, **23**, 26–34.

Symoens, J. and Schuermans, Y., 1979, Levamisole. *Clinics in Rheumatic Diseases*, **5**, 603–629.

Williams, H. J., Ward, J. R., Reading, J. C., *et al.*, 1983, Low-dose D-penicillamine therapy in rheumatoid arthritis: A controlled double-blind clinical trial. *Arthritis and Rheumatism*, **26** 581–592.

7. Corticosteroids

Although the late Nobel Laureate, Dr Philip Hench, of the Mayo Clinic, first speculated, half a century ago, upon the role of the adrenal glands in the aetiology of rheumatoid arthritis, it was not until 1948 that he reported the dramatic beneficial effects of ACTH (corticotrophin) and compounds E (cortisone) and F (cortisol) in rheumatoid arthritis. However, over the next decade, it gradually became apparent that although corticotrophin and oral corticosteroids suppressed joint inflammation, they did not prevent progression of the disease, and had many side-effects. In the late 1950s and early 1960s, carefully conducted therapeutic trials failed to show the superiority of oral corticosteroids over aspirin. Today, it is not fashionable to use corticosteroid therapy in the treatment of rheumatoid arthritis, although it is still used for life-threatening disorders, such as necrotizing arteritis and acute systemic lupus erythematosus, topically for scleritis and for intra-articular injection.

Physiology

Hormonal steroids produced by the adrenal cortex fall into three main categories: The glucocorticoids (principally cortisol or hydrocortisone), which affect intermediate metabolism; the mineralo-corticosteroids (principally aldosterone) which cause the retention of salt and water; and the androgens (principally dehydro-epiandrosterone). Although aldosterone has a purely mineralo-corticoid effect, cortisol also exhibits weak sodium-retaining and androgenic activities.

The normal adrenal secretion of cortisol ranges between 15 and 30 mg/day and there is a pronounced diurnal cycle, plasma concentrations being higher in the morning than in the evening. Cortisol concentrations vary from 5 to 20 μg/dl, approximately 80% being bound to an alpha-2-globulin, corticosteroid-binding globulin or transcortin, synthesized in the liver. Only free cortisol is active. Normally, a small amount of cortisol binds to albumin, although this increases when plasma concentrations exceed 20 to 30 μg/dl, and it is this albumin-bound portion which diffuses into the extravascular fluid. The liver, the major organ responsible for cortisol inactivation, conjugates the reduced products with glucuronic acid to form water-soluble compounds.

The production of cortisol is regulated by corticotrophin released from the anterior pituitary gland. This in turn, is regulated by corticotrophin-releasing factor, produced in the hypothalamus in response to external stimuli such as pyrogens, surgery, hypoglycaemia, exercise and emotional stress. The concentration of free cortisol in plasma has a negative-feedback effect on the higher cortical centres and on the production of both corticotrophin-releasing factor and corticotrophin.

A number of tests are currently employed to assess the integrity of the cerebro-hypothalamo-pituitary-adrenal axis. They are the synacthen test, the metyrapone test, the dexamethasone suppression test and the insulin hypoglycaemia test. Synacthen is a synthetic analogue containing the biologically active N-terminal 1–24 amino acids of naturally occurring corticotrophin. It is widely used as a screening procedure to test adrenal function. However, the feedback regulation of pituitary corticotrophin secretion is best tested by the dexamethasone-suppression test. Metyrapone inhibits the action of 11β-hydroxylase, the enzyme involved in the final stage of cortisol biosynthesis, causing a decrease in plasma cortisol concentration. This promotes the secretion of corticotrophin which stimulates the adrenals to produce inactive 11-deoxycorticosteroid. This can be measured in the form of 17-oxogenic-steroid metabolites, in the urine. An impaired response to metyrapone indicates hypothalamic–pituitary and adrenal hypofunction. The intravenous administration of insulin, to reduce the concentration of blood glucose to less than 50%, causes a marked rise in corticotrophin and cortisol concentrations, and provides a test of the complete hypothalamo-pituitary-adrenal (HPA) axis.

Chemistry

The chemical structure of cortisol and cortisone is shown in figure 7.1. All the glucocorticoids are 21-carbon steroid molecules, and depend for their activity on the presence of four structural features: the ketone on C3, the double bond between C4 and C5, the carbonyl group at position 20 and the hydroxyl group

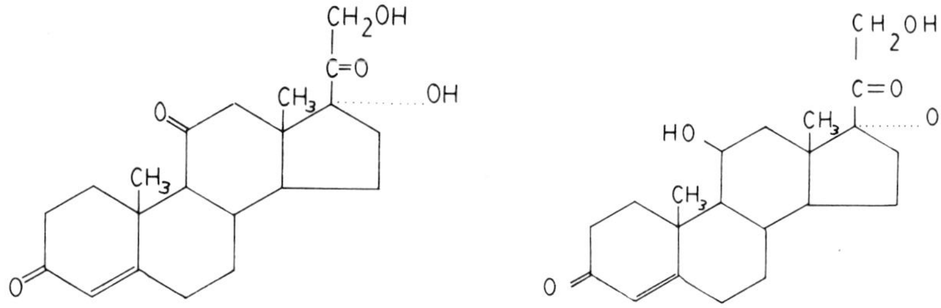

(*a*) (*b*)

Figure 7.1. (*a*) Cortisone and (*b*) cortisol.

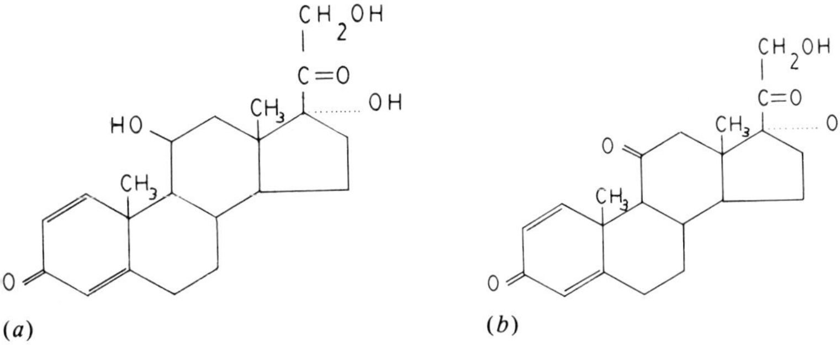

Figure 7.2. (*a*) Prednisolone and (*b*) prednisone.

in the β-position at C11. Cortisone and prednisone, which are 11-keto compounds, must undergo reduction in the liver to their corresponding 11β-hydroxyl compounds, hydrocortisone and prednisolone, before they can become active. Thus, cortisone has no anti-inflammatory effect when injected into an inflamed joint, whereas hydrocortisone has. For this reason, cortisone and prednisone can be regarded as pro-drugs. The structures of prednisone and prednisolone are shown in figure 7.2.

The structural modification and relative glucocorticoid and mineralocorticoid potencies of the commonly used oral corticosteroids are summarized in table 7.1. The duration of anti-inflammatory activity of cortisol and its synthetic analogues closely parallels the duration of HPA suppression. All natural or synthetic corticosteroids possess anti-inflammatory properties and suppress the HPA axis. It is assumed that this is because both the chemical determinants on the steroid molecule, which react with HPA receptors, and those in the peripheral tissues are either the same or are closely related. Unfortunately, improvements in selective pharmacological activity have not been matched by a reduction in multi-system toxicity, except in the case of mineralo-corticoid activity.

Pharmacology

Despite a vast amount of research the mechanism of action of the corticosteroids remains largely unknown. They are, however, known to suppress both cellular and humoral responses. The degree of suppression of inflammation is proportional to the concentration of corticosteroids at the site of inflammation. Thus, their anti-inflammatory action is local. To prevent inflammation the corticosteroids block the permeability of the capillary endothelium reducing the leakage of fluid and the transport of proteins into the area of injury. The exudation of macrophages and other cells is inhibited also, and lysosomal membranes are stabilized. In addition, the reticulo-endothelial clearance of antibody-coated cells is hindered, and prostaglandin production suppressed by

Table 7.1. Structural modifications, relative potencies, and biological half-lives of commonly used synthetic oral corticosteriods.

	Molecular substitutions										
	Double bond	Methyl group									
Preparation	**C1 and 2**	**6α**	**16α**	**16β**	**6α fluoro**	**9α fluoro**	**16α fluoro**	**Glucocorticoid potency***	**Equivalent potency (mg)**	**Mineralo-corticoid activity**	**Biological half-life (hours)**
Cortisol								1	20	2	8–12
Cortisone								0.8	25	2	8–12
Prednisone	+							4	5	1	18–36
Prednisolone	+							4	5	1	18–36
Methylprednisolone	+	+						5	4	0	18–36
Triamcinolone	+					+	+	5	4	0	18–36
Betamethasone	+		+	+		+		25	0.6	0	36–54
Dexamethasone	+		+			+		30	0.75	0	36–54
Paramethasone	+		+		+			10		0	36–54

* Cortisol is arbitarily assigned a value of one
\+ signifies present

the inhibition of arachidonic-acid release from membrane phospholipids. This is a reaction distinct from that of the NSAIDs, which inhibit the cyclo-oxygenase enzyme. Corticosteroids reduce the number of circulating lymphocytes as well, particularly T lymphocytes.

Glucocorticoids have significant effects on carbohydrate, protein and lipid metabolism, stimulating hepatic gluconeogenesis and protein synthesis and inhibiting peripheral tissue synthesis and glucose uptake and use.

Once inside the cell, corticosteroids bind to specific cytoplasmic receptors and pass into the nucleus. The association of the receptor–steroid complex with the chromatin modifies the DNA template and results in an alteration in the rate of synthesis of specific proteins.

Pharmacokinetics

The potency of an oral corticosteroid is related not only to dose, intrinsic potency and plasma elimination half-life, but also to the duration of its biological activity. The biological half-life of a corticosteroid is usually determined by measuring how long the HPA axis is suppressed. Thus, hydrocortisone and cortisone, with biological half-lives of between 8 and 12 hours, are defined as short-acting; prednisolone, methylprednisolone and triamcinolone, with half-lives of 18–36 hours, as intermediate and paramethasone, betamethasone and dexamethasone, with half-lives of 36–54 hours, as long-acting (figures 7.3 and 7.4).

Most glucocorticoids are rapidly absorbed from the gut, but water-soluble esters of cortisol and synthetic-steroid compounds can be administered intravenously to give immediate affect. Minor changes in chemical structure may result in marked changes in the rate of absorption or duration of action of these drugs. The plasma elimination half-life of corticosteroids is relatively short, varying from 90 minutes for cortisol to approximately 180 minutes for prednisolone.

Normally, 90% of the cortisol administered is reversibly bound to plasma proteins (10% bound, by high capacity and low affinity, to albumin and 80%, by high affinity and low capacity, to an α-2 globulin called transcortin). Synthetic analogues of cortisol bind less efficiently to transcortin (approximately 70%) and, as a result, diffuse more completely into tissues. The binding capacity of transcortin is approximately 10–25 μg of cortisol per decilitre of plasma and at cortisol concentrations greater than 25 μg/dl, binding will be largely to albumin. Prednisolone, the most commonly used corticosteroid in clinical practice, shows dose-dependent pharmacokinetics—an increase in dose leading to an increase in volume of distribution and plasma clearance. Diminished albumin concentrations will also lead to higher concentrations of free drug and an enhanced susceptibility to steroid side-effects. Cortisol competitively inhibits prednisolone clearance and plasma protein binding at low (0.075 mg/kg), but not high (1.5 mg/kg), prednisolone doses.

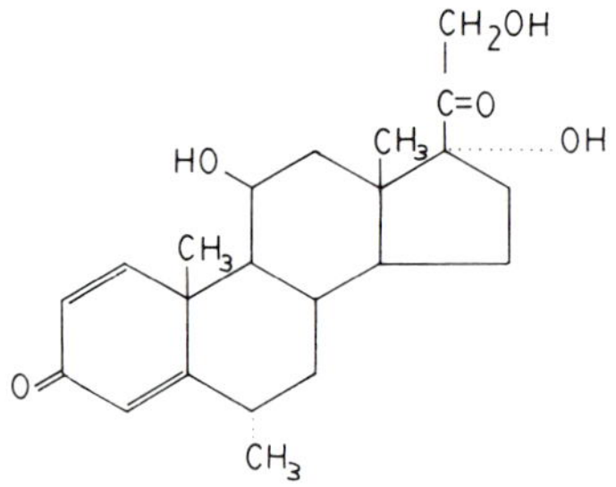

Figure 7.3. 6α-Methyl prednisolone.

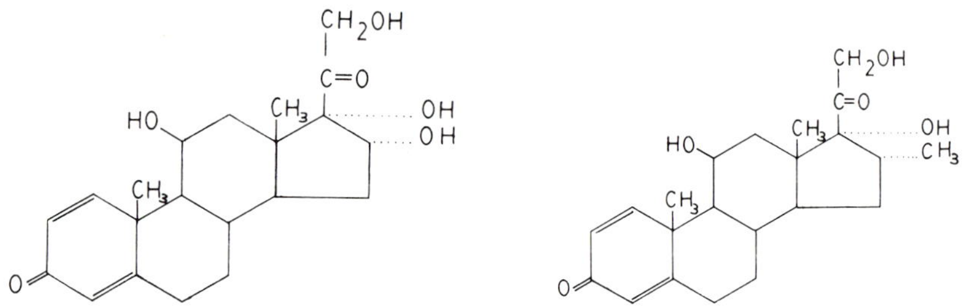

Figure 7.4. (*a*) Triamcinolone and (*b*) dexamethasone.

Gender also affects prednisolone clearance such that female subjects receiving a small dose of prednisolone in the evening have a free clearance approximately 20% higher than males.

Cortisol is rapidly cleared from the circulation by hepatic metabolism and excreted in the urine in the form of inactive glucuronide metabolites. Synthetic analogues of cortisol undergo slower liver metabolism and, therefore, have a prolonged plasma half-life. However, there is marked individual variation in the metabolism of cortisol and the synthetic steroids and, consequently, a wide range of plasma concentrations are seen. Cortisone and prednisone are converted in the liver to their active metabolites, cortisol and prednisolone, a process that can be impaired in patients with liver disease. Nevertheless, there is no apparent relationship between the clinical effect and plasma concentration of cortisol or its synthetic analogues.

Clinical effects

Owing to their low therapeutic ratio, corticosteroids should be prescribed only after careful consideration of the diagnosis and alternative forms of treatment. Once a decision is made to begin corticosteroid therapy, the physician must give the patient clear instructions on compliance with the regime and alert him or her to the possible side-effects. The patient should be provided with a steroid card or preferably encouraged to purchase a 'Medi-alert' bracelet. This is particularly important in young children and the elderly. The overriding principle must be to use the lowest dose possible to control the disease, and for the shortest possible time. Alternate day therapy should be instituted whenever possible in order to minimize side-effects.

When pharmacological doses of oral corticosteroids are required, it is preferable to prescribe synthetic analogues. In most cases, prednisolone still remains the most useful preparation as it does not require hepatic biotransformation to become biologically active. The major disadvantage is that it possesses mineralo-corticoid activity. In clinical practice, however, this problem is largely offset by the range of tablets available (1 and 5 mg). These enable small adjustments in dose to be made and are particularly important when patients are being withdrawn from the drug. An alteration in daily dose such as this cannot be effected with more potent agents such as dexamethasone and betamethasone. For these reasons prednisolone is the corticosteroid of choice for patients with rheumatoid arthritis. Corticotrophin, including depot-tetracosactrin does not offer any therapeutic advantage over oral corticosteroid, and indeed is more likely to produce side-effects such as hypertension and pigmentation.

Weekly or fortnightly injections of methylprednisolone or triamcinolone hexacetonide may be used in patients who cannot comply with oral medication, and a number of clinical trials have supported the use of pulse methylprednisolone therapy. However, while these treatments may be useful in the short term, their long-term efficacy has not been established.

Controlled clinical trials have shown that prednisolone is better than most NSAIDs, in the short term, but there have been no formal trials using low doses (less than 7.5 mg) as an adjunct to other forms of treatment. Recently, it has been suggested that small doses (up to 10 mg) may be useful in maintaining mobility in patients with rheumatoid arthritis without the risk of serious side-effects. Used carefully, corticosteroids are helpful in the management of a number of rheumatic diseases, but their indications for use in rheumatoid arthritis should remain as follows:

1. Acute disease, unresponsive to maximum therapy with NSAIDs, gold, D-penicillamine, hydroxy-chloroquine or immunosuppressive agents. Corticosteroids should not be given without a trial of bed-rest, in hospital.
2. Severe extra-articular disease with evidence of vasculitis of vital organs, scleritis, recurrent pericarditis, diffuse, progressive, pulmonary fibrosis or non-compressive neuropathy.
3. Severe rheumatoid arthritis in the primary financial source of the family, while awaiting therapeutic response to another suppressive agent such as gold, D-penicillamine or an immunosuppressive.

4. For the control of severe progressive disease in patients in whom immobility may be more hazardous than steroid therapy.

The dose of prednisolone should not exceed 10 mg day (in a single morning dose) except in life-threatening circumstances. Once corticosteroids have successfully controlled the disease, attempts at slow dose reduction should be made. On occasions, this has to be carried out at a rate of 1 mg/month, particularly when patients are steroid dependent.

Side-effects

The side-effects of corticosteroid therapy are essentially those of Cushing's syndrome, with suppression of the HPA axis, and even with low doses (10 mg, or less, per day of prednisolone or equivalent) they can be significant.

Oral corticosteroid therapy has been studied extensively in patients with rheumatoid arthritis on long-term low-dose therapy. Suppression first occurs at the hypothalamo–pituitary axis and then at the adrenal glands. However, there is no relationship between the loss of circadian rhythm of plasma cortisol and suppression, and patients with suppression appear capable of a normal adrenal response to surgical stress. Even patients who are incapable of responding to surgical stress by increasing their plasma cortisol, appear not to suffer ill effects. Nevertheless, it is prudent to provide these patients with additional corticosteroid during and after surgery. Surprisingly, there are few well-documented cases of acute adrenocortical insuffiency following chronic oral-corticosteroid therapy. Indeed, the minimal dose of oral corticosteroid required to cause suppression of the HPA axis has not been ascertained and there is no evidence of clinically significant hypothalamo–pituitary suppression in patients receiving long-term corticotrophin therapy.

The recovery of the hypothalamo–pituitary axis is relatively rapid once oral corticosteroid therapy has been withdrawn. On average, the adrenal response to tetracosactrin returns to normal some two weeks afterwards. However, several authors have noted that 12 months are required before the adrenal response to surgical stress returns to normal. Thus, in practical terms, if there is any doubt regarding a patient's ability to respond normally to surgery, it is wise to provide corticosteroid cover.

Withdrawal of corticosteroid therapy, even abruptly, is unlikely to precipitate an Addisonian crisis, but patients may suffer a withdrawal syndrome and their disease is likely to be exacerbated. The use of alternate-day corticosteroid therapy, reduces the suppression of the hypothalamo–pituitary axis as well as the incidence of side-effects and is useful when large doses are required. However, it is often impractical in the treatment of rheumatic diseases because the patients tend to become symptomatic on the non-steroid day. Patients receiving corticosteroids may develop a moon face with facial erythema, truncal obesity, violacious striae, buffalo hump, supraclavicular fat pads, mediastinal widening and rarely, hepatomegaly due to fatty infiltration. At the same time the skin becomes atrophic and the subcutaneous bleeding that results often leads to ulceration. Hyperglycaemia and hyperlipoproteinaemia occur as well. In children, growth is retarded owing to peripheral antagonism of the growth hormone. Corticosteroid therapy induces a negative nitrogen, potassium and calcium balance. The former may accentuate muscle wasting and a distinct myopathy, affecting the shoulder girdle, may develop with the use of fluorinated compounds, such as triamcinolone, dexamethasone and betamethasone. The increased calcium loss in the urine, together with the suppression of calcium absorption from the gastro-intestinal tract and the direct effect on bone metabolism, predispose to osteoporosis and pathological fractures. In rheumatoid arthritis, low-dose corticosteroid therapy causes osteoporosis and aseptic necrosis of the bone, especially the humeral and femoral heads. However, whether calcium supplements, vitamin D, fluoride or oestrogens can minimize these effects remains to be proven.

Low-dose corticosteroid therapy frequently induces a mild euphoria, but does not cause a psychiatric reaction. However, with high doses psychiatric symptoms may develop, especially in individuals with pre-existing psychological problems. Nevertheless, psychological dependence is probably more common than realized. Benign intracranial hypertension occurs in children and should be considered in any patient who develops papilloedema while receiving corticosteroid therapy.

Posterior subcapsular cataracts occur in 5% of patients receiving chronic low-dose corticosteroid therapy, after one year of treatment. The cataracts may become sufficiently large to interfere with vision, and may require surgical removal. Their pathogenesis remains unknown. Both topical- and systemic-corticosteroid therapy may be associated with a rise in intraocular pressure and predispose to glaucoma.

Dyspepsia is a particularly troublesome side-effect, but there is no firm evidence for the development of peptic ulceration. Indeed, it is worth noting that there is no increase in peptic ulceration in spontaneous Cushing's syndrome, or in patients with bronchial asthma or ulcerative colitis treated with corticosteroids. If there is an increased incidence of peptic ulcer in patients with rheumatoid arthritis on corticosteroid therapy then it may be associated with the concomitant use of NSAIDs. Corticosteroid therapy does not reduce the rate of healing of peptic ulcers and there is no evidence that an ulcer that has developed will be more likely to bleed or perforate. However, the clinical features of perforation may be suppressed. There is growing awareness that patients with diverticulitis are more likely to perforate if treated with corticosteroids and, as in the case of perforated peptic ulcer, the clinical features may be suppressed.

Antacids and histamine-blocking drugs are frequently prescribed for patients with dyspepsia caused by corticosteroid therapy, but there is no proof that they control this, or the development of peptic ulceration.

Suppression of the inflammatory response may make the patient more susceptibile to infection and can reactivate pulmonary tuberculosis. Thus, patients with a past history of tuberculosis, need to be reviewed frequently, but routine use of prophylactic anti-tubercular therapy may not be justified in view of the high incidence of hepatic side-effects.

Drug interactions

Corticosteroids may induce the metabolism of salicylates, so that on withdrawal of the former there is a tendency for the concentration of plasma salicylate to rise and cause intoxication. Barbiturates, phenytoin and rifampicin induce microsomal enzymes and as a result, decrease the effect of corticosteroids. Diuretics, except spironolactone and triamterene, have an additive effect on urinary potassium loss, increasing the risk of hypokalaemia. Dexamethasone is less effective if ephedrine is administered along with it, but the mechanism for this has not been established. An interesting interaction occurs with anti-cholinesterase drugs in myasthenia gravis. Corticosteroids improve muscle strength when taken alone, but in combination with anti-cholinesterase drugs they lead to a worsening of symptoms. Of the corticosteroid drugs investigated hydrocortisone is the most potent, followed by prednisolone and methylprednisolone. Strangely, dexamethasone does not exhibit this deleterious effect. Interestingly, oral contraceptives increase the concentration of transcortin, and thus decrease the plasma concentration of free corticosteroid, but there is no evidence that this is of any clinical significance.

Intra-articular and soft-tissue injections and topical use

The intra-articular injection of corticosteroid is a relatively simple and safe exercise, carrying an extremely low risk of post-injection infection. While controlled studies of intra-articular corticosteroids in both rheumatoid arthritis and osteoarthritis suggest an initial benefit, it is unclear how long the effect lasts. Repeated injections, particularly into weight-bearing joints, are not recommended as they may cause or speed joint destruction. Microcrystalline corticosteroid esters may cause the crystal synovitis responsible for a 'post-injection flare'. Certainly, polarized light microscopy of the joint fluid will reveal the presence of weakly positive and/or negative bi-refringent crystals. Cutaneous atrophy at the site of injection has been reported also. This can be delayed in onset and is possibly related to the subcutaneous deposition of corticosteroid. The injection of tendon sheaths needs to be carried out carefully and may be associated with subsequent tendon rupture. The ideal dose of corticosteroid for intralesional injection has not been determined, but as a rough guide in volume equivalents, 1–2 ml is injected into a large joint such as a knee, hip or shoulder, 0.5–1 ml into the ankle or wrist, while small joints

Table 7.2. Steroid preparations available for intra-articular and soft-tissue injection.

Preparation	**Dose (mg/ml)**
Prolonged action	
Prednisolone tertiary butyl acetate	20
Prednisolone pivalate	50
Prednisolone sodium phosphate	16
Methyl prednisolone acetate	40
Triamcinolone acetonide	10–40
Triamcinolone hexacetonide	20
Dexamethasone sodium phosphate	4
Short action	
Hydrocortisone acetate	25
Prednisolone acetate	25

of the fingers usually require 0.1–0.2 ml. A careful aseptic technique should be used while injecting the drug and any excess synovial fluid should be removed before installation. Local anaesthesia is rarely necessary, and there are no controlled data to suggest that techniques such as flushing the needle with sterile saline, to prevent deposition of crystalline material along the tract as the needle is removed, will reduce the incidence of post-injection flare or skin atrophy. While some physicians avoid weight-bearing and reduce activity of the injected joints for 48 hours after intra-articular injection, there is no firm evidence that this minimizes cartilage destruction. The major corticosteroid preparations available for intralesional use are shown in table 7.2.

Patients with psoriatic arthritis may receive a topical corticosteroid preparation such as triamcinolone acetonide cream. However, it is important for the physician to realize that only a small amount of formulation is required for dermatological purposes, since the corticosteroid is absorbed through the skin and may cause suppression of the hypothalamo–pituitary axis and other side-effects.

Topical therapy with ointments and solutions is also used in ophthalmic complications of rheumatic diseases, such as scleritis and iridocylitis. Ocular complications may follow their use including glaucoma, cataracts, visual disturbances, conjunctival petechiae, punctate keratitis, corneal and scleromalacia and infections.

Further reading

Gambertoglio, J. G., Amend, W. J. C. and Benet, L. Z., 1980 Pharmacokinetics and bioavailability of prednisone and prednisolone in health volunteers and patients: A review. *Journal of Pharmacokinetics and Biopharmaceutics*, **8**, 1–52.

Hart, F. D., 1983, Corticosteroid therapy in the rheumatic disorders. In *Antirheumatic Drugs*, edited by E. C. Huskisson (Praeger), p. 497–509.

Meffin, P. J., Brooks, P. M. and Sallustio, B. C., 1984, Alterations in prednisolone disposition as a result of time of administration, gender and dose. *British Journal of Clinical Pharmacology*, **17**, 395–404.

Parrillo, J. E. and Fauci, A. S., 1979, Mechanisms of glucocorticoid action on immune processes. *Annual Review of Pharmacology and Toxicology*, **19**, 179–201.

Pickup, M. E., 1979, Clinical pharmacokinetics of prednisone and prednisolone. *Clinical Pharmacokinetics*, **4**, 111–128.

Swartz, S. L. and Dluhy, R. G., 1978, Corticosteroids: Clinical pharmacology and therapeutic use. *Current Therapeutics*, **19**, 145–170.

8. Immunosuppressive agents

The rationale for using immunosuppressive agents in the treatment of inflammatory joint disease is based upon the belief that immunological activity contributes to joint damage. Over the years a variety of immunosuppressive agents have been used to treat rheumatic disease, but although they have been shown to suppress pain and inflammation in controlled clinical trials, they do not cure the patient and are associated with serious short- and long-term side-effects. The major immunosuppressive drugs used in the rheumatic diseases are shown in table 8.1.

Table 8.1 Immunosuppressive agents used in rheumatic diseases.

Drug	Class
Chlorambucil Cyclophosphamide	Alkylating agents
Methotrexate	Folate antagonist
6-Mercaptopurine Azathioprine	Purine analogues

Alkylating agents

Chlorambucil and cyclophosphamide are the two alkylating agents used in the treatment of rheumatic disease. The alkylating agents undergo strongly electrophilic chemical reactions by forming carbonium-ion intermediates, or by linking with target molecules to form reactive complexes. They link covalently with a variety of biologically important chemical structures including phosphate, amino, sulphydryl, carboxyl and imidazole groups. The cytotoxic activity of the alkylating agents is directly related to the alkylation of DNA. The formation of cross-links within the DNA molecule results in major disruption of its function, leading to both cytotoxic and mutagenic effects.

Alkylating agents may act at any stage in the cell cycle. Toxicity however, is usually only seen when cell division occurs. When these agents induce changes in the DNA strands, repair enzyme systems may act to correct the lesions before the next cell division. If extensive cross-linkage occurs then cell death may result, but minor modifications of DNA structure may not be lethal and may, therefore, be transmitted to the daughter cells.

Chlorambucil

The anti-inflammatory effects of chlorambucil (figure 8.1) have been demonstrated in adjuvant arthritis, although in mycoplasma-induced arthritis, the inflammatory reaction is enhanced. Chlorambucil markedly reduces fibroblast proliferation in animal models of inflammation and reversibly reduces mitosis in bone marrow and lymphoid tissues. It also affects tissues composed of rapidly-dividing cells, such as those found in the reproductive organs and intestinal mucosa. Thus, amenorrhoea and impaired spermatogenesis may occur and damage to the intestinal mucosa may lead to indigestion and diarrhoea. Oral absorption of chlorambucil is rapid and the drug is completely metabolized, having an elimination half-life from plasma of about 90 minutes.

Chlorambucil has been used in one controlled trial and a number of open studies for the treatment of rheumatoid arthritis. Significant improvement in global score was noted in the placebo-controlled study, over a period of three months, and the rheumatoid-factor titre also fell. A clinical response can sometimes be seen within four weeks, but, usually, treatment has to be continued for at least two months before a response is noted. Long-term follow-up studies suggest that only a small percentage of patients remain on chlorambucil after four years. The amount of drug required is from 0.1 to 0.2 mg/kg/day and this can be given as a single dose. After three to six weeks this may be reduced to 2 to 4 mg, depending on clinical improvement or peripheral white-cell count.

The side-effects of chlorambucil are significant with haematological effects (leucopaenia, thrombocytopaenia and anaemia) and secondary infection occurring frequently. Alopecia and amenorrhoea are rare, but there is a marked increase in the incidence of leukaemia and other tumours in patients with rheumatoid arthritis, polycythaemia rubra vera and breast cancer. Thus, it should be reserved for severe cases of rheumatic disease which do not

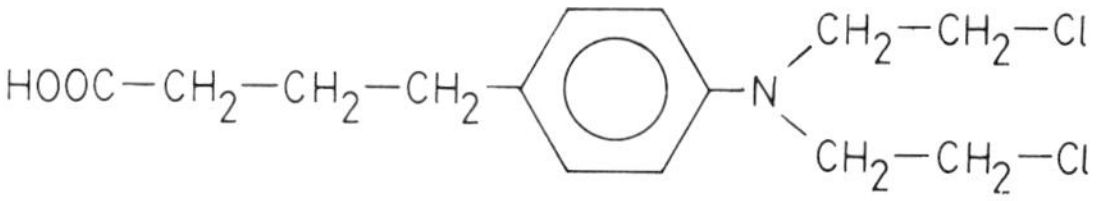

Figure 8.1. Chlorambucil.

respond to other agents and patients should be followed carefully to assess long-term side-effects.

Cyclophosphamide

Cyclophosphamide was designed in an effort to produce a drug which was initially inert, but which could be converted into an active form by dividing cells. Its structure and metabolism is shown in figure 8.2. Cyclophosphamide is readily absorbed from the gastro-intestinal tract and is activated by hepatic microsomal enzymes. Plasma concentrations are achieved one hour after oral administration, and the plasma half-life is about 2–10 hours. The cytochrome P-450 mixed-function-oxidase system in the liver converts cyclophosphamide to 4-hydroxycyclophosphamide which is in equilibrium with the acyclic tautomer aldophosphamide. These compounds can be further broken down to

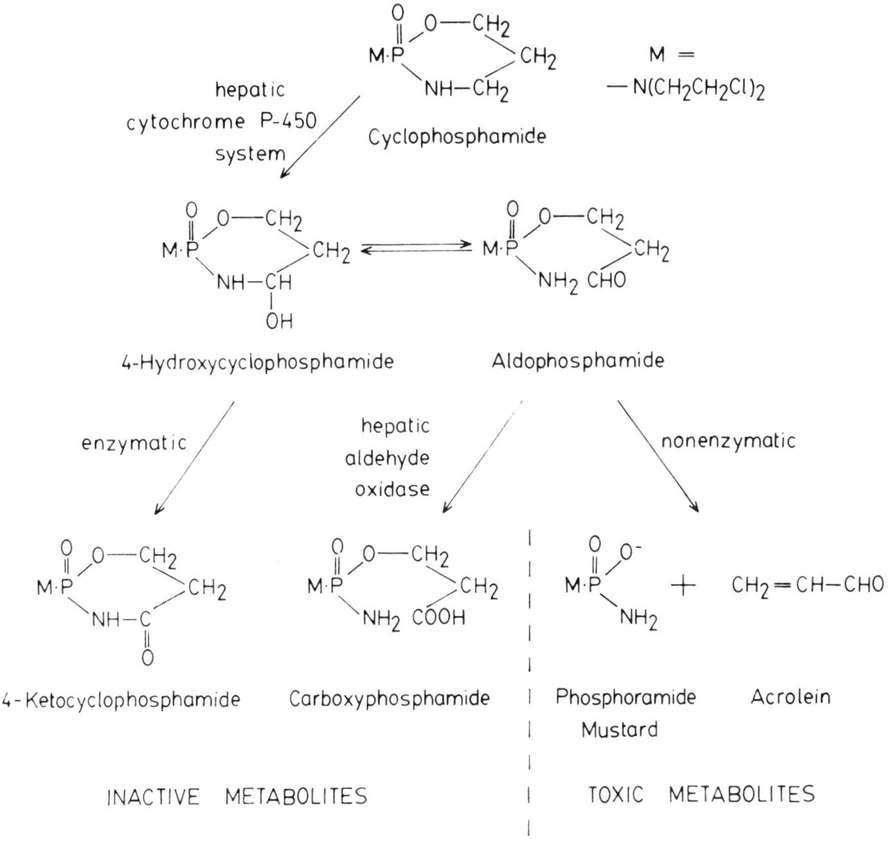

Figure 8.2. Cyclophosphamide and metabolites.

inactive metabolites, or alternatively transported to target sites, where they are converted to the highly toxic metabolites, phosphoramide mustard and acrolein. Urinary recovery of unchanged drug is less than 14%, but metabolites are excreted in the urine and accumulate in patients with renal dysfunction. Cyclophosphamide and its metabolites are both water and lipid soluble and are distributed rapidly throughout the body.

The metabolites of cyclophosphamide have a profound effect on cellular and humoral processes. Transfer of alkyl groups to cellular constituents can alter lymphocyte function, leading to alteration in cell-mediated immunity and antibody production.

In the treatment of severe rheumatoid arthritis, cyclophosphamide is better than a placebo, but the lowest effective dose has not been determined. However, it is known that doses of less than 1 mg/kg/day produce a response that is not significantly different from placebo. A carefully conducted study on 88 patients with rheumatoid arthritis comparing 150 mg/day to 75 mg/day failed to show significant difference, although the side-effects were similar. Cyclophosphamide may be used in combination with low-dose corticosteroid therapy, effectively reducing the dose and toxicity of both drugs. Cyclophosphamide is the current treatment of choice for Wegener's granulomatosis, and possibly for other forms of vasculitis, and can be used in selected patients with rheumatoid arthritis. It has also been used effectively in patients with severe lupus erythematosus or other life-threatening diseases of the connective tissue.

The drug, in common with other nitrogen mustards, inhibits rapidly-dividing, normal, cell populations, leading to bone-marrow depression, alopecia and gastro-intestinal toxicity. Chromosomal abnormalities and teratogenic effects have been found *in vitro* and in laboratory animals. These have also been demonstrated in infants born to mothers with Hodgkin's disease who had been treated with cyclophosphamide during the first trimester of pregnancy. Cyclophosphamide induces sterility and testicular atrophy in males and amenorrhoea with ovarian fibrosis in females. Bladder toxicity, owing to the excretion of toxic metabolites in the urine, is a common side-effect and, although the incidence of this can be reduced, by giving the drug in the morning and providing adequate hydration, continued administration may lead to chronic cystitis. Thus, it has been suggested that intermittent treatment may be more appropriate in patients requiring long-term therapy. This is given monthly in an intravenous bolus. Studics using doses of 0.75 to 1 g/m^2 of body surface area, every three to four weeks, have been used in the treatment of glomerulonephritis, and further studies in rheumatoid arthritis and lupus erythematosus are awaited. Certainly, intermittent therapy reduces the risk of bladder complications and may reduce other side-effects such as alopecia and carcinogenicity.

Cyclophosphamide should be used only for those patients with severe life-threatening disease not responding to other agents. If used orally the dose should be given in the morning with plenty of fluid to reduce the incidence of haemorrhagic cystitis. Careful monitoring of platelet and white-cell counts should be carried out in an attempt to induce a mild leucopaenia (total white-cell count around 3000/mm^3). Cyclophosphamide should be ceased if the total PMN count drops below 1000/mm^3 or the platelet count falls below 100 000/mm^3. In patients undergoing long-term treatment, consideration should be given to intermittent bolus treatment using intravenous therapy (0.75 to 1 g/m^2 of body surface area) every three to four weeks. Since cyclophosphamide is activated by liver enzymes, great care should be taken in patients treated with other liver enzyme inducers or inhibitors, for example, barbiturates or corticosteroids, and close monitoring for side-effects should be undertaken.

Folate antagonists

Methotrexate

Methotrexate (figure 8.3) is a folic-acid antagonist which is used increasingly for the treatment of rheumatic disease. It interferes with the enzyme dihydrofolate reductase, which is responsible for the conversion of folates to their active, reduced form. The depletion of intracellular reduced-folate concentrations leads to the inhibition of thymidylate and purine production, which effectively blocks the synthesis of RNA and DNA. As well as inhibiting both DNA and RNA synthesis, methotrexate may also interfere with protein synthesis and cell growth can be interrupted during both the "S" and "G" phases of the cell cycle. As with the folates, methotrexate is extensively metabolized to polyglutamate derivatives, which can remain within the cell for long periods of time. It is possible that polyglutamate formation plays a role in the production of the long-term side-effects of methotrexate, including hepatic fibrosis and renal toxicity. Polyglutamate derivatives inhibit dihydrofolate reductase and are cytotoxic.

The rate of absorption and total bioavailability of methotrexate after oral administration shows marked variability between patients and is dependent on the dose administered. Bioavailability is significantly reduced at the high doses (in excess of 50 mg/m^2) used to treat neoplastic disease. In the smaller doses employed for the treatment of rheumatic disease (10 to 20 mg total dose) it is almost completely absorbed. Peak plasma concentrations occur 1 to 5 hours

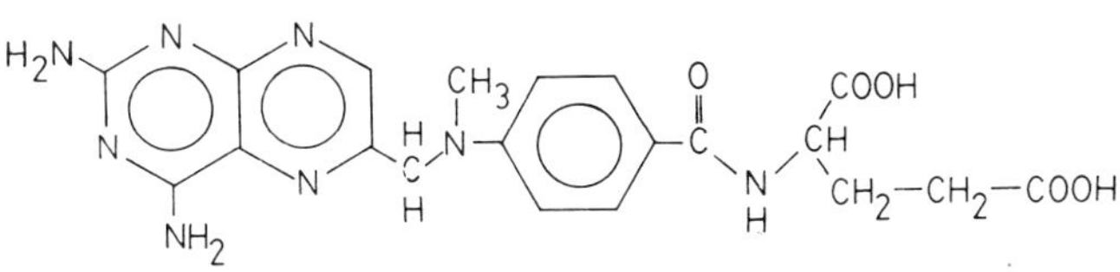

Figure 8.3. Methotrexate.

after oral administration and the drug is excreted primarily by the kidneys. In man, the disposition is triphasic with the final phase being in excess of 27 hours. Extensive enterohepatic recycling, and enteric bacterial metabolism also occurs. Methotrexate is strongly bound to plasma proteins and may be displaced by a variety of NSAIDs. Aspirin and other NSAIDs, being weak organic acids, reduce the renal excretion of methotrexate, adding to the potential for serious interaction. However, although agranulocytosis has been described with the concurrent use of salicylate in patients with neoplastic disorders, no such problems have been reported in patients with rheumatic disorders treated with methotrexate and NSAIDs.

Experience with low-dose methotrexate has now been reported in rheumatoid arthritis, psoriatic arthritis, polymyositis and Reiter's syndrome. Several open studies have reported the effects of a weekly dose of methotrexate given, intra-muscularly or orally, to patients with rheumatoid arthritis. These have shown the suppression of disease activity, but an incidence of side-effects comparable to other immunosuppressive agents. More recently, a collaborative trial carried out by the American Rheumatism Asssociation has shown that methotrexate, in doses of 15 mg weekly, is significantly better than a placebo over a 16-week period. The optimal dose of methotrexate has not yet been determined, but a small clinical study has shown no difference between the use of 25 mg and 10 mg methotrexate per week, although both were significantly better than a placebo over a 12-week period. Further trials are required to assess its full potential. A number of side-effects have been reported with methotrexate in addition to marrow toxicity. These include pulmonary fibrosis, renal impairment, hepatotoxicity and sterility. Although it is clear that hepatotoxicity can be reduced by intermittent dosing, gastrointestinal symptoms and abnormalities of liver function are still common. It has been suggested that patients receiving cumulative doses of methotrexate in excess of 1.5 g should be subjected to liver biopsy, but at present there is no clinical evidence to support this. Nevertheless, all patients on methotrexate should be followed carefully for evidence of long-term hepatoxicity and carcinogenesis.

Purine analogues

6-Mercaptopurine and azathioprine

These drugs are purine analogues, which inhibit a variety of enzymes necessary for DNA and RNA synthesis. The exact mode of action of these drugs is unknown, although there is evidence of a wide range of biochemical effects, directed at DNA, RNA and purine nucleotide synthesis. 6-Mercaptopurine (6-MP) is absorbed rapidly after oral ingestion and about 50% of the dose is excreted via the urine within 24 hours. It has a plasma half-life of about 90 minutes, owing to renal excretion, uptake by cells and metabolism, and is

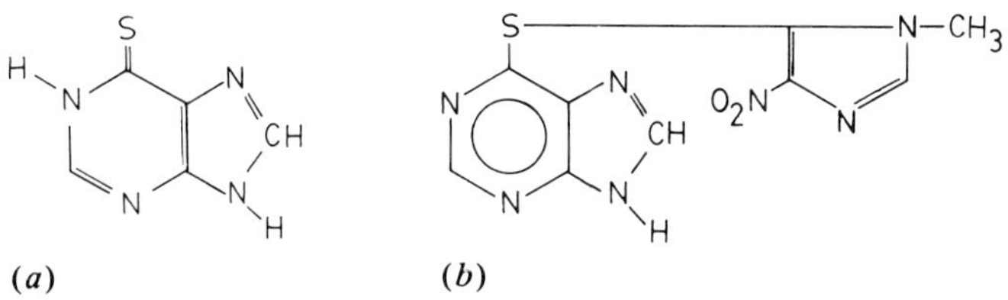

Figure 8.4. (*a*) 6-Mercaptopurine and (*b*) azathioprine.

metabolized along two major pathways, one involving the methylation of the sulphydryl group and subsequent oxidation, and the other producing 6-thiouric acid after oxidation by xanthine oxidase. This latter pathway is significantly reduced by allopurinol, the concurrent administration of which will significantly increase both the immunosuppressive and toxic effects of 6-MP and azathioprine.

The structures of 6-MP and the imidazole derivative azathioprine are shown in figure 8.4. Azathioprine is metabolized *in vivo* to yield 6-MP. Azathioprine has long-term efficacy, compared with a placebo, gold, cyclophosphamide and D-penicillamine, in the treatment of severe rheumatoid arthritis. It slows the rate of radiological progression of rheumatoid arthritis and reduces corticosteroid dependency. No clearly significant differences have been shown in these comparative studies, but azathioprine is perhaps easier to use than cyclophosphamide. Substitution of a placebo, in patients whose disease has been suppressed by long-term azathioprine, results in clinical deterioration, indicating the need for long-term therapy. The optimal dose of azathioprine has yet to be determined, but a dose of 1.25 mg/kg/day would seem to be as efficacious as 2.5 mg/kg/day and it is therefore suggested that the patient be commenced on between 1–1.25 mg/kg/day; the larger doses being reserved for those patients who do not respond within three months of therapy. Side-effects are common with azathioprine, but are not usually serious. Nausea and vomiting and other gastro-intestinal disturbances occur frequently and occasionally hepatitis or pancreatitis develop. Leucopaenia is common, but the suspension of therapy usually results in a rapid recovery. As with other immunosuppressive agents, long-term side-effects, particularly carcinogenesis, may be of significance. There are conflicting data as to whether patients with rheumatoid arthritis are more likely to develop tumours, but immunosuppressive therapy following renal transplantation is known to be associated with an increased incidence and further studies are required to fully assess the risks and benefits of azathioprine in the treatment of rheumatic disease.

From the practical point of view, patients receiving azathioprine require careful medical supervision in order that adverse drug reactions are detected and appropriately treated before they become severe. A full blood count should be carried out each month and the patient warned to return to the physician if unexpected problems arise. Azathioprine causes sterility and should be avoided in young patients and pregnant women. However, it can be useful in patients with severe rheumatoid arthritis or systemic lupus erythematosus.

A recent study comparing azathioprine and D-penicillamine in a large group of patients with rheumatoid arthritis over a 24-week period has shown evidence of an improvement in both groups. Differences between treatments were not clinically significant though there were fewer adverse reactions in patients receiving azathioprine.

Further reading

Barnes, C. G. and Lovatt, G. E., 1982, Modifying the disease process in rheumatoid arthritis: immunosuppression in perspective. *Annals of the Rheumatic Diseases*, **41**, (Supplement 1) 1–60.

Chabner, B. A., Myers, C. E., Coleman, C. N. and Johns, D. G., 1975, Clinical pharmacology of anti-neoplastic agents. *New England Journal of Medicine*, **212**, 1107–1113.

Groff, G. D., Shenberger, K. N., Wilke, W. S. and Taylor, T. H., 1983, Low-dose oral methotrexate in rheumatoid arthritis: an uncontrolled trial and review of the literature. *Seminars in Arthritis and Rheumatism*, **12** (4), 333–347.

Jolivet, J., Cowan, K. H., Curt, G. A., Glendeninn, N. J. and Chabner, B. A., 1983, The pharmacology and clinical use of methotrexate. *New England Journal of Medicine*, **309**, 1094–1104.

Kirwan, J. and Currey, H. L. F., 1984, Rheumatoid arthritis: disease modifying anti-rheumatic drugs. *Clinics in Rheumatic Diseases*, **9**, 581–588.

Kovarsky, J., 1983, Clinical pharmacology and toxicology of cyclophosphamide. Emphasis on use in rheumatic diseases. *Seminars in Arthritis and Rheumatism*, **12** (4), 359–372.

Paulus, H. E., Williams, H. J., Ward, J. R. *et al.*, 1984, Azathioprine versus D-penicillamine in rheumatoid arthritis patients who had been treated unsuccessfully with gold. *Arthritis and Rheumatism*, **27**, 721–727.

9. Drugs used in gout

Gout is a form of arthritis induced by deposition of monosodium urate crystals in joint tissues. Joint inflammation results from the local infiltration of granulocytes, which phagocytose the crystals and stimulate the release of a variety of inflammatory mediators. Crystal deposition is a consequence of excess urate within the body, although local factors appear to play a part in the acute event.

Elevated levels of uric acid arise either because there is overproduction by the body or there is under-excretion, although both mechanisms may occur together. Increased production may be the result of a genetically-controlled enzyme deficiency or a consequence of myeloproliferative disorders, high purine intake, alcohol consumption or obesity and hypertriglyceridaemia. Reduced excretion of uric acid may be genetically determined or secondary to renal disease, hypertension, drugs (diuretic agents and low-dose salicylates), lactic acidosis or a low volume of urine.

Gout can be treated as an acute attack, chronic disease or asymptomatic hyperuricaemia. Treatment of the acute attack requires potent anti-inflammatory agents such as colchicine or an NSAID. Most NSAIDs are effective, although relatively high doses (e.g., up to 300 mg of indomethacin can be taken in the first 24 hours) must be used. If the attack persists, oral or intra-articular corticosteroids may be used. Once the acute attack has been controlled, the use of drugs capable of lowering the concentration of uric acid must be considered. Two groups of drugs can be used, either the xanthine-oxidase inhibitors, such as allopurinol, which reduce uric acid production, or the uricosuric agents which increase renal excretion. Drugs which alter uric acid concentration in blood should not be used during an acute attack. Where patients are suffering from recurrent attacks of gout, or where major organ damage due to deposition of uric acid is present, (e.g. renal stones or urate nephropathy) urate-lowering drugs should be used. However, the treatment of asymptomatic hyperuricaemia is less clear. The patients with hyperuricaemia risk the development of gouty arthritis, renal disease, hypertension and vascular disease. While the association between raised serum-urate concentrations and gouty arthritis is clear, the relationship between uric acid and renal disease, hypertension and vascular disease is less well defined. There is little

Table 9.1 Drugs used in gout.

Colchine
Non-steroidal anti-inflammatory drugs
Xanthine-oxidase inhibitors
Allopurinol
Uricosuric agents
Probenecid
Sulphinpyrazone
Benzbromarone
Azapropazone
NSAIDs
Diflunisal

evidence to support treatment of mild (<0.6mmol/l) asymptomatic hyperuricaemia. Patients with uric acid concentrations in the range 0.42–0.6 mmol/l should be reviewed frequently for evidence of renal disease, vascular disease, hypertension and gout, but generally do not require treatment for hyperuricaemia. The drugs used in the management of acute gout and hyperuricaemia are shown in table 9.1.

Colchicine

Colchicine (figure 9.1) is an alkaloid, derived from the autumn crocus, or meadow saffron (*Colchicum autumnale*) and has been used throughout history for the treatment of aches and pains. It may inhibit the chemotaxis of neutrophils by interfering with microtubule assembly and with phagocytosis. There is some evidence that colchicine also prevents production or release of pro-inflammatory substances from neutrophils. It has no effect on the concentration of serum uric acid.

Colchicine is rapidly absorbed after oral administration with peak concentrations occurring within two hours. Considerable entero-hepatic recycling occurs and the drug can still be detected in leucocytes about 10 days after a single intravenous dose. Metabolism occurs in the liver and most of the drug is excreted in the faeces. The plasma half-life is less than one hour although

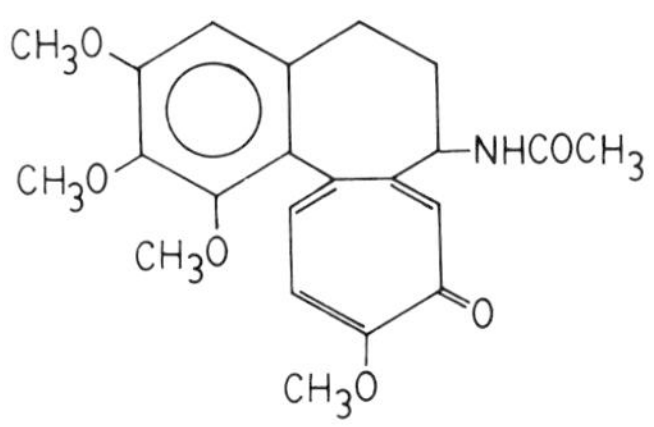

Figure 9.1. Colchicine.

colchicine reaches stable concentrations in leucocytes, of about 10 times the plasma concentration for up to 24 hours. After absorption, colchicine metabolism occurs in the liver, but methodological problems have precluded metabolite studies in man. Colchicine is excreted primarily in the faeces and although 20% is excreted in the urine, no dose modification needs to be made in patients with mild to moderate renal function undergoing short courses of treatment.

Although controlled clinical trials have not been conducted, there seems little doubt from open studies that colchicine reduces the duration of the acute attack as well as attacks in patients controlled with uricosuric agents. These studies have formed the basis of the use of colchicine as a prophylactic in a dose of 1–2 mg/day. The toxicity of colchicine is dose-related and varies with the route of administration. Following oral administration, gastro-intestinal toxicity is common, particularly diarrhoea, although abdominal cramps, nausea, and vomiting can also occur and haemorrhagic gastroenteritis has been observed in cases of overdose. These side-effects can sometimes be reduced by giving the drug intravenously, but care must be taken with the injection as it can cause local tissue necrosis and cardiotoxicity. The risk of toxicity is increased in patients with chronic liver disease and death has been described following doses as small as 7 mg. Occasionally, haematological complications occur with disseminated intravascular coagulation, bone-marrow failure and thrombocytopaenia.

In the prophylaxis of gouty arthritis, colchicine should be prescribed in a dose of 0.5 mg two or three times per day. Since the drugs that alter uric acid concentration may precipitate gout attacks when first administered, colchicine should be prescribed for a period of three months. In the treatment of acute gouty arthritis colchicine may be used as an alternative to NSAIDs. It is customary to prescribe 1 mg initially and then 1 mg orally every two to three hours until relief is obtained or side-effects occur. If patients have not responded by the time they have received a total of 6 mg, a NSAID should be used. For intravenous use 1–2 mg of colchicine is dissolved in 20 ml of saline and given by slow infusion. The dose may be repeated if a response does not occur with four to six hours.

Xanthine-oxidase inhibitors

Allopurinol

Allopurinol (figure 9.2), an analogue of hypoxanthine, was first synthesized as a therapeutic agent for use in leukaemia. It inhibits xanthine oxidase, blocking the conversion of 6-thiopurine to 6-thiouric acid. Both allopurinol and its major metabolite, oxipurinol are analogues of hypoxanthine and xanthine, respectively and are potent inhibitors of xanthine oxidase. The administration of allopurinol leads to a decrease in the concentrations of plasma and urinary

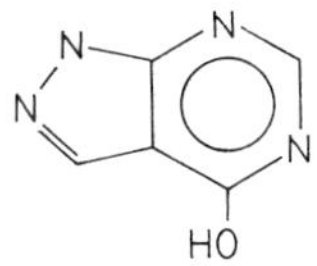

Figure 9.2. Allopurinol.

uric acid. It also interferes with a variety of other metabolic pathways, including pyrimidine biosynthesis, tryptophan pyrrolase and purine nucleoside phosphorylase.

Allopurinol is rapidly absorbed after oral ingestion and peak concentrations are found in the plasma within one hour. Approximately 20% of the drug is excreted in the faeces within 72 hours. It is rapidly cleared from the plasma, primarily by conversion to oxipurinol, and has a half-life of two to three hours. This conversion is dose-dependent, with 10% of a single dose, or 30% a chronic dose, being excreted unchanged in the urine. The half-life of oxipurinol is much longer than that of allopurinol (18–30 hours) and its excretion is dependent on renal function. Although oxipurinol is a less potent inhibitor of xanthine oxidase than the parent compound, the accumulation of oxipurinol during chronic administration contributes significantly to the therapeutic effect. Both allopurinol and oxipurinol are widely distributed in body water and neither is significantly bound to plasma proteins.

Allopurinol is effective in lowering uric-acid concentrations in both the hyperuricaemia of primary gout and that secondary to polycythaemia vera and other blood dyscrasias. The administration of allopurinol to patients with normal renal function is followed within 48 hours by a decrease in the concentrations of serum and urinary uric acid. The maximum reduction occurs within two weeks and remains fairly constant after that time. In most patients concentrations of serum uric acid can be reduced to normal on a dose of 300 mg/day, but the occasional patient will require up to 1000 mg/day. Owing to the prolonged half-life of the biologically-active oxipurinol, a once daily dose is appropriate. Resolution of tophi will occur during prolonged therapy and the progression of gouty nephropathy appears to stop in most patients. Once allopurinol therapy has started and the serum urate has been reduced to normal concentrations, the lowest dose required to maintain those concentrations should be employed. Although it is thought that, once commenced, drug therapy should be continued indefinitely, there is some evidence to suggest that after a period of time allopurinol can be withdrawn without the recurrence of gouty arthritis.

Serious toxicity is rare and only about 5% of patients have to cease treatment. Allopurinol is associated with gastro-intestinal intolerance, thrombocytopaenia, vasculitis and skin reactions. The total incidence of side-effects is about 20% and they are more likely to occur in the presence of renal insufficiency. Skin rashes are the most frequent serious side-effects and are more common in patients receiving concurrent therapy with thiazide diuretics or ampicillin. Occasionally it may be necessary to consider desensitizing patients who have had skin rashes if no alternative treatment for the reduction of uric acid exists. Xanthine stones in the kidney and oxipurinol crystal deposition in the muscle have occasionally been reported in patients with very high uric acid excretion. Acute attacks of gouty arthritis are common on initial treatment with allopurinol and patients should be protected with colchicine or an NSAID during the first three months of therapy.

Drug interactions are frequent, the most serious being those with the purine analogues azathioprine and 6-mercaptopurine. Indeed, the dose of azathioprine or 6-mercaptopurine should be reduced to 30% of that usually administered if the patient is receiving allopurinol as well. The elimination half-life of probenecid is increased 50% by allopurinol and the toxicity of other cytotoxic agents, such as cyclophosphamide, appears to be enhanced, although the mechanism is unclear. As allopurinol and oxipurinol affect microsomal enzymes in the liver, it is necessary to reduce and monitor the dose of oral anti-coagulants if allopurinol therapy is to be administered concurrently. Allopurinol can be given in an initial, single dose of 100 to 300 mg/day of uric acid, but the plasma urate should be checked at regular intervals to ensure that this is adequate. Patients should be encouraged to maintain a good volume of urine and prescribed colchicine or an NSAID during the first three months of therapy.

Uricosuric drugs

Probenecid

Probenecid was developed in an effort to prolong the efficacy of penicillin by reducing its rapid renal excretion. Probenecid is a lipid-soluble benzoic acid derivative whose structure is shown in figure 9.3. It inhibits the transport of organic acids across epithelial barriers, particularly in the renal tubule, where it inhibits the tubular resorption of filtered uric acid. Probenecid also inhibits the tubular secretion of penicillin, salicylates, dapsone and a variety of other weak organic acids.

Probenecid is rapidly absorbed following oral administration and strongly bound to plasma proteins (in excess of 90%). The elimination half-life of

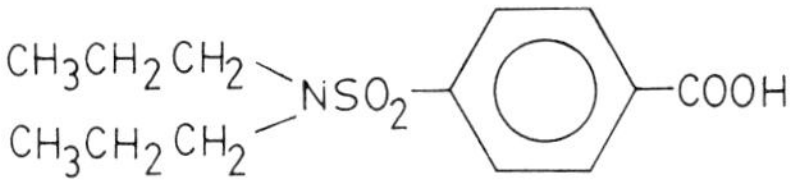

Figure 9.3. Probenecid.

probenecid in plasma is dose-dependent and ranges from 6 to 12 hours. It is rapidly metabolized and its major glucuronide metabolite is excreted in the urine. Some of the hydroxylated urinary metabolites also have uricosuric activity.

Probenecid is usually given in a dose of 1–2 g/day. Therapy should be initiated slowly, over a period of 1–2 weeks, to avoid the sudden excretion of large quantities of uric acid and the risk of crystalluria. Fluid intake should be encouraged during this stage and the urine should be made alkaline. Most patients can achieve a satisfactory concentration of serum urate on 1.5 and 2 g/day. Approximately 10% of them will suffer gastro-intestinal side-effects, and, occasionally, hypersensitive skin rashes occur.

Probenecid influences the renal excretion, volume of distribution and hepatic uptake of a number of other drugs. It reduces the renal excretion of salicylates, dapsone, sulfinpyrazone, indomethacin and the penicillins. A reduced volume of distribution of antibiotics, such as ampicillin, nafcillin, and cephaloridine, has been noted, while probenecid also decreases the hepatic uptake and metabolism of ampicillin, indomethacin, naproxen, ketoprofen and diflunisal and causes some prolongation in metabolism of heparin. The uricosuric action of probenecid is itself blocked by the salicylates.

Probenecid should be commenced in a dose of 0.5 g/day with fluid loading and alkalinization of the urine. The daily dose can be increased, after three to four days, to 1 to 2 g. Serum urate should be checked at regular intervals and prophylaxis against acute attacks of gout using colchicine or an NSAID during the first three months of treatment.

Sulfinpyrazone

Sulfinpyrazone is a pyrazole derivative, chemically related to phenylbutazone (figure 9.4). It is a potent inhibitor of the tubular resorption of uric acid and reduces the renal excretion of other organic anions. Sulfinpyrazone lacks the anti-inflammatory activity of its congener phenylbutazone, but reduces platelet aggregation and prolongs platelet survival.

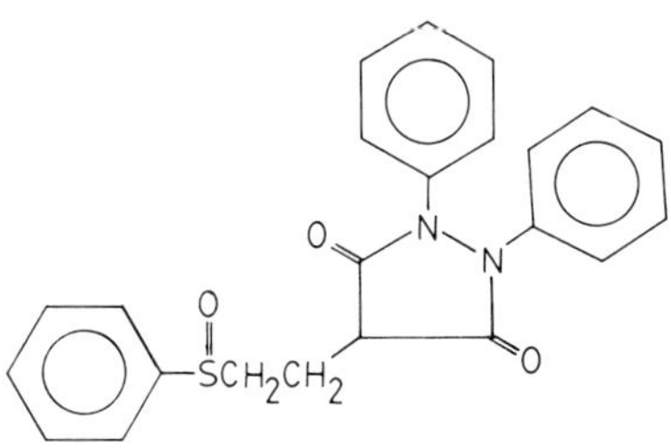

Figure 9.4. Sulfinpyrazone.

Sulfinpyrazone is rapidly absorbed after oral administration and is strongly bound to plasma proteins (98%). Owing to this, its distribution is largely confined to the extracellular space. Sulfinpyrazone has a plasma half-life of approximately three hours, but its uricosuric effect may last for up to 10 hours. Some of the drug is excreted unchanged in the urine, the remainder being metabolized by the liver and eliminated as a hydroxyphenyl; a potent uricosuric agent also.

The normal maintenance dose of sulfinpyrazone ranges from 300 to 400 mg/day and can be prescribed twice daily. It should be introduced slowly over a period of three weeks and the dose increased until the desired concentration of serum uric acid is achieved. As with probenecid, a high fluid intake and alkalinization of the urine is important during the first months of therapy. The major side-effects of sulfinpyrazone are gastro-intestinal and they occur as frequently as those of probenecid.

Benzbromarone

Benzbromarone (figure 9.5) is a relatively new uricosuric agent. Although it has been shown to be a weak inhibitor of xanthine oxidase *in vitro*, there is no suggestion that this is responsible for its effect in man.

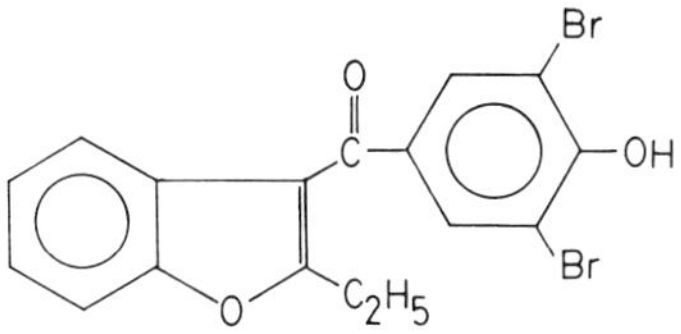

Figure 9.5. Benzbromarone.

Benzbromarone is rapidly absorbed from the gut and is metabolized to monobromine and dehalogenated derivatives, both of which have uricosuric activity. The elimination half-life of benzbromarone is in the range of six to eight hours, but the effect on uric acid excretion lasts for much longer, allowing for once daily administration.

The usual dose of benzbromarone is 40–80 mg/day and similar guidelines apply to its administration as to other uricosuric agents. The concurrent use of salicylate with benzbromarone does not interfere with its uricosuric activity, as it does with other uricosuric agents, suggesting that benzbromarone may act at a different site in the renal tubule than probenecid or sulfinpyrazone. The drug has not been widely used and side-effects have not been extensively reported.

NSAIDs

The NSAIDs, being acidic, may have weak uricosuric effects. This is particularly marked with compounds such as diflunisal and azapropazone and is seen over a wide dose range, although low doses of some NSAIDs may lead to uric acid retention.

Principles of uricosuric use

Uricosuric agents have an important role to play in the treatment of hyperuricaemia and gout, but like all drugs need to be used carefully. Their efficacy is reduced in patients who have renal insufficiency and an increased dose is necessary to achieve satisfactory hypouricaemia. The use of uricosuric agents is contra-indicated in patients with over-production of urate or high urinary urate; a past history of renal calculi; a persistently poor urine volume; a past history of sensitivity to these drugs; and those currently suffering an acute attack of gouty arthritis.

In treating patients with hyperuricaemia and gout, other factors, such as diet and other medications, which might increase serum urate should always be investigated before commencing drug therapy. Patients require careful instruction as to the importance of maintaining an adequate urine volume and their concentrations of serum uric acid should be monitored at frequent intervals to ensure compliance.

Further reading

Emmerson, B. T, 1983, *Hyperuricaemia and Gout in Clinical Practice* (Adis Health Science Press).

Kelley, W. N. and Holmes, E. W., 1985, Anti-hyper-uricaemia drugs. In *Textbook of Rheumatology*, Edited by W. N. Kelley, E. D. Harris, S. Ruddy, and C. B. Sledge, (W. B. Saunders) 2nd edition, p. 857–871.

Meyrier, A., 1976, Desensitisation in a patient with chronic renal disease and severe allergy to allopurinol. *British Medical Journal*, **2**, 458.

Wallace, S. L., 1974, Colchicine. *Seminars in Arthritis and Rheumatism*, **5**, 369–381.

Index